Expressway to FATMD Listening Test

全国医学博士英语统考
听力一本通

主　编　蒋　跃

副主编　曹扬波　李　娟　周俊佑

编　者　刘书凝　杨天元　张英贤　沈音序
　　　　吴　鸽　余碧燕　吕豆豆　于　群

人民卫生出版社
·北　京·

图书在版编目（CIP）数据

2024 全国医学博士英语统考听力一本通 / 蒋跃主编
. —北京：人民卫生出版社，2023.12

ISBN 978-7-117-35871-2

Ⅰ. ①2… Ⅱ. ①蒋… Ⅲ. ①医学－英语－听说教学
－博士生入学考试－自学参考资料 Ⅳ. ①R

中国国家版本馆 CIP 数据核字（2023）第 243879 号

人卫智网	www.ipmph.com	医学教育、学术、考试、健康，购书智慧智能综合服务平台
人卫官网	www.pmph.com	人卫官方资讯发布平台

2024 全国医学博士英语统考听力一本通

2024 Quanguo Yixue Boshi Yingyu Tongkao Tingli Yibentong

主　　编：蒋　跃
出版发行：人民卫生出版社（中继线 010-59780011）
地　　址：北京市朝阳区潘家园南里 19 号
邮　　编：100021
E - mail：pmph @ pmph.com
购书热线：010-59787592　010-59787584　010-65264830
印　　刷：三河市国英印务有限公司
经　　销：新华书店
开　　本：850×1168　1/16　　印张：15
字　　数：454 千字
版　　次：2023 年 12 月第 1 版
印　　次：2024 年 1 月第 1 次印刷
标准书号：ISBN 978-7-117-35871-2
定　　价：79.00 元

打击盗版举报电话：010-59787491　E-mail：WQ @ pmph.com
质量问题联系电话：010-59787234　E-mail：zhiliang @ pmph.com
数字融合服务电话：4001118166　E-mail：zengzhi @ pmph.com

2024 版序

金风送爽，丹桂飘香。中秋国庆佳节之际，我们共同迎来了经过修订的《2024 全国医学博士英语统考模拟试题》(简称《模拟试题》)和《2024 全国医学博士英语统考听力一本通》(简称《听力一本通》)的付梓。这是我们连续 24 年为广大医学博士考生奉献的辅导教材，也是您备战医学博士英语统考不可或缺的伴侣和助手。

在过去的 23 年里，秉承着服务考生和着眼实战的初心，我们始终致力于提供高质量的考博英语辅导教材。在 2024 版的修订工作中，我们全力以赴、精心打磨。我们深知，平时的英语学习、复习，以及阅读量的积累是提高考试成绩的关键。因此，我们通过精选优质习题和详细解析的方式，助力考生更好地掌握医学博士英语统考的考点和技巧。

这里简述一下 2024 版两本书的修订情况。一是对 2023 版中发现的一些错误和疏漏进行勘误和补充。二是在《听力一本通》中增加了一套根据 2020 年新考试大纲命题的高仿真试题。三是根据近两三年来的真题和考试情况，替换了部分写作内容。比如，我们在 2024 版的《模拟试题》中增加了一套翻译题及对其的解答和答题技巧。四是对听力进行了部分修订和录音重新灌制。值得一提的是，为了让考生能够适应各种不同的英语口音、语速和音质，我们在录音灌制过程中邀请了多位口音和音质不同的外籍教师参与，通过反复审听和调整，使得录音的质量得到了明显提升，也提高了录音的多样性。我们深信，这将为您的听力训练带来更好的效果，提高您在听力考试中的应变能力。2024 版两本书的总修订量将近 35%。

最后，我想向编写团队、出版社编辑及每一位读者表示由衷的感谢。正是有了大家的参与、支持、使用和反馈，这两本书才能不断地得到完善和改进。您的信任是我们最大的动力，也是我们不断前行的方向。

古人诗云："银烛秋光冷画屏，轻罗小扇扑流萤。"秋天的美妙，总是让人心生诗意。在此，我附上打油诗一首，以表我对考生的祝福：

> 金秋时节红叶飞，丹桂芬芳夜霜微。
>
> 医路漫漫梦探寻，英语复习伴吾身。
>
> 岁月如梭光阴逝，修订新篇彰辉煌。
>
> 编者群英用心笔，考生支持我长久。

让我们一同携手迎接新版《2024 全国医学博士英语统考模拟试题》和《2024 全国医学博士英语统考听力一本通》的到来，继续痛并快乐着的英语学习旅程，砥砺前行！

祝各位考博顺利。

蒋 跃

2023 年中秋节于梧桐西舍

目 录

Part I Strategies for Listening Comprehension

医学博士英语统考听力考试高分策略

2020 年初，国家医学考试中心公布了全国医学博士英语统考的最新考试大纲，对听力和书面表达的考试内容和题型进行了修改。至此，2020 年医学博士英语统考迎来了自 2002 年以来，18 年后的第一次题型改革。到 2024 年，考试大纲修订已经 4 年了，但对很多初次参加全国医学博士英语统考的考生和读者来说，还是有必要在这里对最新考试大纲中的听力进行理解。这一部分大致描述如下：

听力考试时间（录音播放英语的时间）约为 28 分钟，分为两部分：Section A 为 5 个小对话（mini-conversations），每个对话约 100 个词，含 3 道题，题型包括主旨概括、具体细节、判断推理，共计 15 题和 15 分，内容涉及医患对话、保健、文化、学生日常生活的各个方面，其核心内容是各种各样的医疗、学习、生活情景；Section B 为 5 个片段（mini-talks），每个片段约 150 个词，含 3 道题，题型包括主旨概括、具体细节、判断推理，共计 15 题和 15 分，所谈话题一般为挂号、预约、健康、疾病、治疗、学习、生活等内容，大都涉及医学内容，也有一些话题跟医学毫无关系；片段由 1 人（或男或女）朗读，或以教师讲课模式，或以电视或广播录音模式，或以读一段文字的形式，内容涉及文理科各个专业的内容，尤以医学科普内容为多，难度相对较大，但一般不会很专业化。关于医学博士听力常考的内容，我们用八个字来概括："医普、文化、生活、学习"。

听力部分含两种题型，各为一节（Section）。

Section A: 对话（Conversations）

这一部分一改 2002 年以来一直沿用的 15 个短对话的题型，改成了共 5 个 mini-conversations 对话，每个对话各 3 道小题，共计 15 题，15 分；每个对话约 100 个词，旨在测试考生对英语对话的听力理解能力，考点分别为：①主旨概括；②具体细节；③判断推理。通常情况下，主旨概括都位居每个对话题中的首位，其余两个考点一般都会出现。与其他英语考试（如大学英语四、六级考试及 TOEFL）新题型中听力的对话部分题型类似，只是题数不同和有些医学内容而已。

Section B: 短文（Passages）

这一部分题型也有变化，不是过去的 1 个长对话加 2 个片段，而是 5 个片段，各 3 道小题，共计 15 题，15 分；每个片段约 150 个词，旨在测试考生对英语篇章的听力理解能力。要求考生回答每篇短文所附的 3 个问题。这一节与其他英语考试听力题型大同小异，但其特点是都含有与医学相关的内容或题材。

往届试题里，医学题材或内容的比例是 1/2，从 2012 年起几乎每年的试题中都有两个短文与医学有关。在医学博士英语统考中，听力是大家感觉相对较难、准备周期较长的一部分。这些考生大多从事临床医学工作多年，脱离外语学习时间很久，最擅长做词汇、完形填空和语法题，对于听力往往都是"谈虎变色"，心中没底。其实，世间万物各有其律，听力也有很多规律可循。从开始准备考试起，就应该有针对性地在听力方面多下一些功夫，寻找其中规律性的东西。实际上，在 FATMD 考试中，听力分数的高低往往决定了总分的高低。

如何较快地提高听力应试水平呢？本文将结合听力考试的两个部分及近几年试题的变化思路谈谈

相应的对策。

一、对话题(Section A: Conversations)复习要点

1. 多练听抄,逐字琢磨回味

所谓"听抄",就是听写,就是拿一段听力录音来反复播放,哪怕是一个单词都可以反复播放,直到琢磨出来并抄下来为止,不到万不得已不查看原文。

这里推荐一个听抄软件,叫 Cool Edit,网上有这个软件的免费版,Windows 解压安装后就可以使用。用户也可以网上购买下载"Adobe Audition CC 20××"app,其使用界面与 Cool Edit 是一样的。它最大的好处就是可以随意定位想听的录音,让考生想听哪个部分的听力,甚至哪个音节,都可以听,而且还可以反复多遍地定点播放某一个单词、短语、句子,或者句子片段,随时停顿下来抄写,直至听懂。

最后再核对原文(script)。这是恢复听力的最快、最有效的方法。当然,这需要考生踏踏实实,逐字逐句地听写之后才核对。这个核对过程也是个很重要的学习过程。恍然大悟之间,考生会明白正确和错误的原因之所在,语感也会越来越好。这个做法有几个好处:

1)迅速提高语感;

2)熟悉内容形式;

3)加速听力恢复;

4)克服心理恐惧。

很多考生反映这个方法对他们听力的提高极为有效。

2. 体会医学及各种生活学习思维,熟悉情景及相关词汇

医学博士听力考试的重点内容是医学、健康、生活、学习的方方面面,所以做题时一定要体会医生、患者及学生的思维,把对题目的理解置于医院、医疗、健康、校园等背景中去。例如,平常的医患或健康方面的对话中,无非就是预约看病、头疼脑热、体检、查房、病案讨论等;学生生活中,最为关心的无非就是考试分数、老师严格与否、教授讲课是否有趣等。如:

M: After his accident, doctors gave Ben little chance of surviving, much less of playing golf professionally again.

W: It's incredible that Ben was back on the golf course again within 18 months.

M: What is known about Ben 18 months after the accident?

通常听力考试简短对话部分的核心是一个个的生活情景,而常考的生活情景数量是很有限的。综合各类考题中的简短对话可以发现,其中并没有出现太多的新情景。所以,对于考过的情景一定要进一步细化,弄清其基本规律,记住其中的关键词。例如,医学博士听力中可能常常谈到预约看病,此时首先要注意听看病的场合对不对,在选项中找"appointment, schedule, prescription, nurse, reception room, wait"等字样;考试是听力部分的热门话题,在大多数情况下,题中都会说谁又没有及格,很难过什么;或者说这家伙活该,因为他不够刻苦等,所以会说"You should have studied harder";又比如在噪声情景中,喜欢考"A 没有意识到自己已经打搅了 B"这样的内容,而后面的建议一般是调低音量,因此要注意听诸如"didn't realize, turn down"等关键词。

综上所述,在准备考试的过程中,最好把以前见过的或英语老师提到或总结过的常见情景及例题认真复习,熟悉并掌握其规律,特别是要熟记各个情景常考的关键词。这一点可以参见这本书后面的三个词汇表,分别是,"Part Ⅳ. 临床病历表格常用术语、Part Ⅴ. 常用听力词汇表、Part Ⅵ. 医学英语词汇表"。

3. 提高心理素质,控制做题节奏

大多数同学在考试中不同程度地存在着"**慢热**"、"**走神**"和"**预读选项速度慢**"等方面的问题。这些问题在一定程度上与心理素质有关。因此,在平时的复习和练习中要注意培养磨炼心理素质,控制做题节奏,这样才能克服上述三种问题。下面分别介绍克服这三种问题的方法。

"**慢热**"是指有的同学开头几道题总是错误较多,迟迟进入不了考试状态,听不进去。这种问题可以通过两种方法解决：①多次设置模拟环境，进行模拟考试，平时训练时在时间方面严格要求自己；② Well beginning is half done。考试中一拿到考卷，马上集中注意力预读前三四题的选项，对这几题的内容进行预测。这样可以使你在开头的几道题中做到心中有数。前几道题连续做好了，信心就会越来越足。但预读的选项不要太多，读得再多也记不住，还不如把开头做好。

"走神"是考生普遍存在的问题。Section A 的第 4～5 个对话，Section B 的第 4～5 个片段中，容易"魂不守舍"。这是由这几个部分一般题数较多和听力考试时间到了最后阶段造成的。每次考试，要听的内容实际时间长度只有 20 分钟左右（监考指令和各部分的指令考生通常都耳熟能详，一般都不听）。所以，在平时练习时，最好一次不间断地听题超过 30 分钟，或者一次听 1～2 套整题。只有每次练习的时间长度都超过实际考试听题的长度，才能有效地避免走神的情况。另外，预读选项也可以帮助克服走神的问题。

"预读选项速度慢"也是需要练习的一个环节。很多时候，虽然题听懂了，但由于读选项的速度跟不上，造成选择错误。建议大家有意识地练习选项（关于解决"慢热"的方法中也曾提到），对每一个选项要像阅读一样快速地读一遍。阅读中找出选项中的**异同点**，注意选项中的多音节词和听力中较为生僻的词，这些词往往可能出现在录音当中。复习的时候着重比较正确选项和自己所选择的错误选项之间的差异，体会命题选项设计上的一些陷阱。

另外，不要忘记听力考试中题与题之间的间隔只有短短的 10～12 秒钟，所以考试中一定要控制好做题节奏。个别难题听不懂要舍得放弃，不要在某一道题上花费过长的时间，要抓紧预读下一道题的选项。听力部分首先要争取把自己会做的题都做对，所以，保持平和的心态是至关重要的。

4. 熟记常考习语，注意各种音变

医学博士听力考试是标准化考试，因此具有规律性和重复性的特点。尽管 FATMD 听力中的简短对话与新大纲之前的题型相比是新题型，但对多数考生来说在以往的四、六级，托福及研究生考试复习过程中，可以发现很多的习惯用语多次出现，有的甚至出现十多次。例如"You can say that again"（再说一遍也不会错）、"It serves you right!"（你活该！）、"You're telling me!（还要你告诉我！我早就知道了！）"等等都多次在试题中出现。在复习中，考过的习语也会重复出现，同一习语在不同情景中是可以通用的。如"I dozed off halfway"这个句子，第一次可能是问教授讲课有没有意思，当然是没意思了，而后来这个句型又先后用来评价电影和报告，其意思自然也是"无聊，没劲"。因此，建议大家把本书后面所列的常见的习语认真复习，因为其中任何一个都可能在一次考试中出现。

两个以上单词构成的习语，其发音必然会发生变化，会出现包括连读、失去爆破、弱化等各种音变，使原本熟悉的单词听起来也会觉得陌生。下面几个例子中的习语就可以说明这一点：

I can't **get rid of it.**

The work **has walked Tom off his legs(feet).**

最好的办法：把书后面的常见习语好好地朗读一遍。所以，对于听力部分的单词和习语，一定要养成开口念的习惯，在朗读中熟悉各种音变，这样才有可能在考试中准确地分辨它们。另外，书中还有关于如何辨认语音上容易混淆的词语的分项练习。

5. 分析典型语气，跟读听力原文

目前多种英语听力考试的简短对话在新增情景不多的情况下，语气题的分量开始增加，而且多以难题的形式出现。比如转折语气，就已经成为每套题必考的项目，而且数量一般还不止一道。如：

W: Now, Mr. Cross, don't hesitate to help yourself to some more potatoes, vegetables or roast beef.

M: It's been a wonderful dinner, but if I eat another bite, I think I'll burst.

W: What will the man do?

请注意第二句中间的 but，这是转折语气的标志。所以一般在小对话第二句中如果出现 but，考试重心必然落在 but 后面的转折语气上。不信试试看：找出任何一套题来，看看此类题型的数量。

对于语气题，大家在多听的同时一定要跟读，养成跟着录音朗读的习惯，尽量跟上朗读的速度，并模仿语音和语调。各种听力考试中喜怒哀乐的语气正是在不断跟读和模仿中揣摩出来的。

二、片段题（Section B: Passages）复习要点

1. 多练听抄，逐字琢磨回味

片段题同对话题一样，也需要"多练听抄，逐字琢磨回味"，怎么强调也不过分。方法同前，略。

2. 把握主题大意，注意选项关系

片段题的最大特征就是重点考查对于片段主题大意的理解，这一点集中体现在选项长度明显加长、细节题考得相对较少及大多数片段的几个正确选项在逻辑上都有密切联系等方面。听片段时，一定要注意整体性。不论该片段听得多么吃力，中间有多少处没有听懂，都应该强迫自己把余下的部分听完。不要过分在乎片段中某个具体细节或者句子是否听懂，只要主题大意听明白了，几个问题做对了，目的就达到了。

片段题正确选项之间的逻辑关系一般很紧密，出题也是按短文或对话的时间先后顺序设计的。有些答案其实可以通过分析得出。例如有一个片段谈失眠的问题，上一道题问是什么原因造成的（工作太晚、晚上活动剧烈等引起），下一道题问会导致什么后果（血压升高、情绪急躁等）。由此可见，正确选项相互之间的逻辑关系非常清晰。

3. 听好开头、结尾，同义替换才是解

新大纲规定，Section B 片段或长对话的每个片段都有 3 个问题。这 3 个问题的分布通常都很均匀：开头一道（主旨概括），结尾一道（细节或者判断），中间一道（细节或者判断）。所以每个片段的开头和结尾特别重要，直接影响到对原文全文的理解。这跟阅读理解片段比较类似。与对话题稍有不同的地方是，对话题是"听到什么不选什么"，而不是以"同义替换是解"为主，而片段题最重要的做题原则之一便是"听到什么选什么"或称"原词作答"。所谓"原词"，即片段中重复频率最高或特别强调的某一个词，从语气上是可以听出来的。因此，片段开头要听好"开头原词"，结尾要听好"结尾原词"。对于那些专业色彩较浓的片段，这一原则尤为有效。包含这种原词的选项一般都是正确答案。例如有一个讲解压力的片段，整个片段都在重复 stress 和 anxiety 两个词，那么包含这两个词的两个选项一般就是正确选项。当然，到底是以"同义替换才是解"为主还是"听到什么选什么"，要根据出题情况而定，不能一概而论，考生读者需要灵活掌握和运用。

4. 注意常见套话，记住固定结构

很多片段都有一些固定的套话和引子，用来表达强调、解释、比较、因果等关系。如在讲课类片段中，老师喜欢这样开头"I'd like to begin my first lecture by introducing…"或"Today we will focus on…"，这时，本次课的主题便成为必考问题；下课时老师喜欢说"We'll continue with this next time"或"Your assignment today will be…"，这时，问题一般涉及下次上课的时间或内容；而上课过程中老师喜欢说"Remember to…"或"You are required to…"，这些被强调的地方也会是考点。所以在听完一个片段后务必要记住常用的一些套话和固定结构。

5. 横听同类片段，体会段子规律

听力中有一些片段话题经常被考到，比如各种新的疗法、风俗习惯对疾病的影响、医患对话、看病预约、讨论病情或健康话题，或考试、选课、打工、实习等内容，所以把同一类型的片段放在一起听很有益处，可以比较好地掌握其中的规律。比如疾病片段中必谈疾病的症状、病因和治疗手段，谈文化必然谈国内外风土人情，实习片段中必谈实习任务和学生感受等。

总之，医学博士听力考试中医学内容是必不可少的，对此要做相应的准备。又如某些片段中可能会出现关于异国他乡的风土人情等内容，环境保护和节约能源等方面的内容也是近年来的热门片段类型。

三、本书使用方法

1. 新大纲，新题型，新材料，新录音

针对 2020 年新版考试大纲和 2020 年以来的 5 次真实考试，今年这一版的一本通对听力材料进行

了全部更新,全部重新命题和语言测试与评估(信度、效度、难度等指标)。对测试题答案的呈现和解释也进行了改革。比如,将每个问题的答案都标注在了每套题的听力原文文本当中,相关答案出处在原文中用下划线标出,这样就省掉了大量的文字解释,而是让读者能直接到原文中寻找答案,而不是孤立地撇开原文去看中文解释,更加方便读者学习。

2. 有规律,有计划,有针对性

在使用本书时,要注意讲究方法。比如,①可以结合蒋老师在辅导班上所发材料中没有听力题的练习套题,拼接出一套模拟考试题;②可以摘出 1～2 套用于练习听抄;③听抄过的内容可以随时播放用来磨耳朵,熟悉语音语调和考试内容与形式(比如常见的提问方式)等。

四、其他听力材料的选择

听力考试的准备时间,一般以 2～3 个月为佳。在两个多月的准备过程中,建议大家以本作者主编的两本书中的听力部分为主,而且要本着"好钢用在刀刃上,新题放在最后听"的原则。由于精力所限,不必在其他的听力材料上花太多的时间。但从长远考虑,要在各类听力,尤其是医学博士听力考试中取得高分,还是应该适当补充一些其他听力材料,使自己具备超出医学博士听力考试所要求的水平。可以选择的材料包括各类托福听力材料和模拟试题、真题;蒋跃主编的历年《全国医学博士英语统考模拟试题》、《全国医学博士英语统考听力一本通》(即本书);原文电视录音(补充生活习语),如《急诊室的故事》(E.R.)。建议大家尤其要精听电影原文录音,因为它可以弥补我们在生活情景和日常句型这两个方面的不足。另外,像《英语 900 句》等口语教材也会有所帮助。总之,不管补充什么材料,都应以"真题为主"。

医学博士考试固然重要,固然艰难,但对每个考生来说,这只是学术生涯和人生道路上要迈过的众多门槛之一。所以,无论是在平时还是在考试时,都要有一颗平常心。否则,精神压力太大会严重影响听力考试时的发挥。

最后,祝大家考试顺利。

Practice Test 1

PAPER ONE

Part I Listening Comprehension (30%)

Section A

Directions: *In this section, you will hear five conversations. At the end of each conversation, you will hear three questions about the conversation. The question will be spoken only once. After you hear the question, read the four possible answers marked A, B, C, and D. Choose the best answer and mark the letter of your choice on the **ANSWER SHEET**.*

Sample Answer
A B ● D

Listen to the following example.

You will hear:

   W: Can you tell me about yourself, please?

   M: Sure, my name's Harry, 18 years old, currently studying biology and chemistry at school. As you are aware, I hope to pursue a career in medicine.

   W: Harry, why do you want to be a doctor?

   M: Well, everyone in my family is a doctor, so I think I can follow on nicely. (2. A)

   W: Apart from treating patients, what do you think being a doctor is going to require?

   M: Well, you also need to be academic and have to be an excellent communicator (3. B) with your team and the patients.

Question No. 1: What are the two speakers talking about?

You will read:

1.   A. Switching to biology and chemistry.
     B. Choosing to be a family physician.
     C. Going to college.
     D. **Being a doctor.**

*The correct answer is D. Mark the right answer on the **ANSWER SHEET** as indicated below:*

1.A B C ●

Question No. 2: Why does Harry choose to be a doctor?

You will read:

2.   A. **Because of his family influence.**
     B. Because of the fact that he's young.
     C. Because of the practical skills he has.
     D. Because of his love for biology and chemistry.

*The correct answer is A. Mark the right answer on the **ANSWER SHEET** as indicated below:*

2. ● B C D

Question No. 3: What is mentioned by Harry as one of the requirements for a doctor?
You will read:

3.　A. A strong sense of responsibility.

　　B. **Good communicative skills**.

　　C. Excellent health.

　　D. Great patience.

The correct answer is B. Mark the right answer on the **ANSWER SHEET** *as indicated below:*

3. A　●　C　D

Now let's begin with Conversation One.

Conversation One

1.　A. Patient privacy and data security.　　B. Potential biases in AI algorithms.

　　C. Lack of policies and regulations.　　D. Accountability in critical decisions.

2.　A. They can jeopardize patient safety.

　　B. They hinder technological advancements.

　　C. They lead to legal complications.

　　D. They prioritize certain patients over others.

3.　A. Protocols and regulations are necessary for openness and liability.

　　B. For openness and liability, protocols and regulations must be legalized.

　　C. They disagree on the need for policies and regulations.

　　D. They doubt the need to hold AI accountable for important decisions.

Conversation Two

4.　A. Their different educational backgrounds.　　B. Changing attitudes toward nature.

　　C. Chaos theory and its applications.　　D. The current global economic crisis.

5.　A. Stockbroker.　　B. Physicist.

　　C. Mathematician.　　D. Economist.

6.　A. Improve computer programming.　　B. Explain certain natural phenomena.

　　C. Predict global population growth.　　D. Promote national financial health.

Conversation Three

7.　A. Different kinds of music.　　B. The singer's musical habits.

　　C. The singer's experience.　　D. Different ways to write songs.

8.　A. Touch his heart.　　B. Make him cry.

　　C. Remind him of his life.　　D. Make him feel young.

9.　A. Go to a bar and drink for hours.　　B. Go to an isolated place to sing blues.

　　C. Go to see a performance in a concert hall.　　D. Go to work and wrap himself up in music.

Conversation Four

10.　A. How news-subs write stories.　　B. How news-subs mark sad stories.

　　C. How the man prepares for his work.　　D. How the man refines news stories.

11.　A. They write the first version of news stories.　　B. They gather news stories on the spot.

　　C. They polish incoming news stories.　　D. They write comments on major news stories.

12.　A. Reading through the news stories in a given period of time.

　　B. Having little time to read the news before going on the air.

　　C. Having to change the tone of his voice from time to time.

　　D. Getting all the words and phrases pronounced correctly.

Conversation Five

13. A. Borrowing calculator.
    C. The steel sheets.
    B. The penalty clauses.
    D. Delayed delivery of the control desks.

14. A. To inform him of a problem they face.
    B. To request him to purchase control desks.
    C. To discuss the content of a project report.
    D. To ask him to fix the dictating machine.

15. A. By marking down the unit price.
    C. By allowing more time for delivery.
    B. By accepting the penalty clauses.
    D. By promising better after-sales service.

Section B

Directions: *In this section, you will hear five passages. At the end of each passage, you will hear three questions about the passage. The question will be spoken only once. After you hear the question, read the four possible answers marked A, B, C, and D. Choose the best answer and mark the letter of your choice on the* **ANSWER SHEET**.

Sample Answer

A　B　●　D

Passage One

16. A. Enough replacement of body fluid.
    C. Enough carbonated drinks.
    B. Enough rest before vigorous exercise.
    D. Enough warm-up exercise.

17. A. Graceful.
    C. Rhythmic.
    B. Energetic.
    D. Melodious.

18. A. Drink eight ounces of fluid every ten minutes.
    B. Drink four ounces of water every twenty minutes.
    C. Drink eight ounces of liquid every twenty minutes.
    D. Drink whenever you feel thirsty.

Passage Two

19. A. The poisonous effect of lead in house paint.
    B. The uses of lead in modern America.
    C. The method of locating leads in paints.
    D. The importance of providing universal education.

20. A. Any house.
    B. An apartment building that hasn't been restored in 30 years.
    C. A painting.
    D. A recently painted house.

21. A. In a classroom.
    C. In a paint-making factory.
    B. In a hospital.
    D. In a radio program.

Passage Three

22. A. The importance of time.
    B. The American manager's story.
    C. The cultural difference.
    D. Different meanings of parts of the day in different cultures.

23. A. 10:00 a.m.
    C. 2:00 a.m.
    B. 12:00 a.m.
    D. 2:00 p.m.

24. A. To have a talk with him.
    B. To inform him of their decision.
    C. To discuss a problem with him.
    D. To tell him a problem they met with.

Passage Four

25. A. The side effects of the Heimlich manoeuvre.
    B. The causes of death in choking cases.
    C. What choking is like.
    D. How to use the Heimlich manoeuvre into the abdomen.

26. A. A slow depression of the ribcage.
    B. Repeated thumps on the back.
    C. A quick upper thrust into the abdomen.
    D. An application of force below the belly button.

27. A. A choking victim is best treated in a hospital.
    B. A person who is choking can help himself.
    C. The Heimlich manoeuvre is a recent development.
    D. Choking victims are rarely confused with heart attack victims.

Passage Five

28. A. How thermographic photography was invented.
    B. Scientific photography for diagnostic purposes.
    C. The advantages of X-rays over thermography.
    D. Several new techniques for reducing pain.

29. A. With charts and graphs.
    B. With a thermometer.
    C. With different colours.
    D. With moving lights.

30. A. It is not painful.
    B. Patients can use the pictures.
    C. The process is very relaxing.
    D. No radiation is involved.

Stop   **Stop**   **Stop**

模拟答题卡

姓　　名

准考证号

报考学校

填涂说明　　正确填涂 ●　　错误填涂 ⊘ ⊗ ⊖ ⊜

缺考违纪标记栏：　缺考 ○　　作弊 ○　　（此项由监考人员填涂！）

考生须知

1.答题前，考生务必用黑色字迹签字笔或水笔将姓名、准考证号、报考学校填写清楚。
2.按照题号顺序在各题目的答题区域内作答，未在对应的答题区域作答或超出答题区域的作答均不给分。
3.选择题用2B铅笔作答，不得使用涂改液。

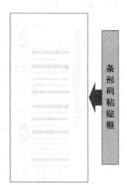

条形码粘贴框

选择题									
1	(A)	(B)	(C)	(D)	16	(A)	(B)	(C)	(D)
2	(A)	(B)	(C)	(D)	17	(A)	(B)	(C)	(D)
3	(A)	(B)	(C)	(D)	18	(A)	(B)	(C)	(D)
4	(A)	(B)	(C)	(D)	19	(A)	(B)	(C)	(D)
5	(A)	(B)	(C)	(D)	20	(A)	(B)	(C)	(D)
6	(A)	(B)	(C)	(D)	21	(A)	(B)	(C)	(D)
7	(A)	(B)	(C)	(D)	22	(A)	(B)	(C)	(D)
8	(A)	(B)	(C)	(D)	23	(A)	(B)	(C)	(D)
9	(A)	(B)	(C)	(D)	24	(A)	(B)	(C)	(D)
10	(A)	(B)	(C)	(D)	25	(A)	(B)	(C)	(D)
11	(A)	(B)	(C)	(D)	26	(A)	(B)	(C)	(D)
12	(A)	(B)	(C)	(D)	27	(A)	(B)	(C)	(D)
13	(A)	(B)	(C)	(D)	28	(A)	(B)	(C)	(D)
14	(A)	(B)	(C)	(D)	29	(A)	(B)	(C)	(D)
15	(A)	(B)	(C)	(D)	30	(A)	(B)	(C)	(D)

书面表达　请用黑色签字笔在答题区域内作答，超出边框无效！

Detailed Explanations of Answers to Practice Test 1

Part I   Listening Comprehension—Tapescript and Answer Keys

Section A

Conversation One (Word count: 109)

W: Hey Eric, we really need to talk about the ethical stuff surrounding AI in healthcare.

M: What specific problems are you talking about?

W: Well, some doctors are freaking out about the potential biases in AI algorithms. (1. B)

M: Ah, got it. That makes sense. Biased algorithms could totally lead to unfair treatment.

W: Exactly. But we also need to think about patient privacy and keeping their data safe. (2. A)

M: Absolutely. AI systems better be rock-solid when it comes to protecting sensitive information.

W: And here's another thing-what about holding AI accountable for important decisions?

M: Oh yeah, we definitely need some policies and rules to make sure transparency and responsibility are in place. (3. A)

   1. What is the primary ethical concern discussed by the two speakers?   B)（主旨概括）

   2. Why are the two speakers concerned about biased algorithms in AI?   A)（具体细节）

   3. Which of the following best reflects the speakers' position on the matter?   A)（判断推理）

Conversation Two (Word count: 108)

M: Kathy, chaos theory seems to be a branch of physics or mathematics. You are an economist, so how does it influence your work? (5. D)

W: Well, in several ways. I am responsible for financial development programs in many parts of the world, so forecasting long range trends and making predictions on the basis of present evidence is what I do. Chaos theory was developed by scientists, trying to explain the movement of the planets and the changes in environmental conditions. (6. B) Both of these things are also about making long-term predictions on the basis of present evidence.

M: Are many economists involved in this field?

W: An increasing number.

   4. What are the speakers mainly talking about?   C)（主旨概括）

   5. What is the woman's profession?   D)（具体细节）

   6. What was chaos theory supposed to do when it was first formulated?   B)（判断推理）

Conversation Three (Word count: 109)

W: Charles, as a singer, do you ever make yourself cry when you sing?

M: No, not at this age. I'm an old man. But the songs can still get through to me. (8. A)

W: What's the most difficult kind of music to sing?

M: It depends. If I like something, I can sing it.

W: Can you perform music that's out of tune with the mood you might be in on a given night?

M: Yes. If my personal life is hurting, I can go to work and the music will take over. It's like a guy who goes to a bar and drinks. For those few hours, I can wrap myself up in my music. (9. D)

   7. What are the speakers talking about?   B)（主旨概括）

   8. What does Charles say songs can do when he sings them?   A)（具体细节）

   9. What would Charles do when his personal life is hurting?   D)（判断推理）

Conversation Four (Word count: 116)

W: I wonder if you could tell me a little bit about your job as a radio announcer.

M: Well, in the news room I am sitting with reporters and news-subs.

W: Sorry, what do you mean by "news-subs"?

M: They are sub-editors. They are the people who write the news stories as they come in. (11. A) I have a chance to read through most stories before I go on the air. Sometimes things happen at the last moment and I don't have a chance. So I've just got to do my best, and take a couple of seconds to look through the first few lines before I launch into something. (12. B)

W: There is nothing to mark what is out of entity?

M: No. If it's something sad, I'll put a small cross at the top.

10. What is this conversation mainly about?	C)（主旨概括）
11. What does the man say news-subs do?	A)（具体细节）
12. What does the man say is a big challenge for him?	B)（判断推理）

Conversation Five (Word count: 122)

W: John. Can I borrow your calculator?

M: Of course. But can you spare me a second? It's the message you sent me about the delivery delay of the control desks. (14. A) What's gone wrong?

W: Everything. Well, the suppliers have got some trouble. They will be late with the delivery.

M: But they can't. The desks are a special order wanted for one of the big computer companies.

W: When did we promise the delivery?

M: Thursday next week. And there's a penalty clause. We stand to lose 10% of our price for each week of overdue delivery.

W: Oh, these penalty clauses! Why did you sales people accept them?

M: We have to accept them; otherwise, we don't get the contracts. (15. B)

13. What is the conversation mainly talking about?	D)（主旨概括）
14. Why did the woman send the message to the man?	A)（判断推理）
15. How did the man get the contracts?	B)（具体细节）

Section B

Passage One (Word count: 143)

The aerobic dance this class is about to introduce is vigorous. (17. B) Before we begin this dance, I would like to give you some hints about how to keep from running dry during vigorous exercise.

Supplying the equivalent fluid you lose during exercise can enhance your performance and diminish the heat stress. (16. A) Don't just wait until you are thirsty. Thirst is a poor indicator of how much fluid you need because by the time you feel thirsty you might already be dehydrated, and you might not be sure of how much you need to drink to meet your body's fluid requirement. It's very important that you replace enough water while exercising during this class, especially if you sweat heavily. Here are the tips:

First, drink water before the class.

Secondly, drink about eight ounces of water or fruit juice every twenty minutes during the class. (18. C)

16. According to the speaker, which of the following elements will improve one's performance?

A)（主旨概括）

17. The type of dance this class is introducing can best be described in which of the following ways?

B)（判断推理）

18. Which of the following is the closest to the suggestion the teacher gave?　　C)（具体细节）

Passage Two (Word count: 154)

Today, our series on "Chemicals in the Household" will focus on lead poisoning. (19. A) The term "lead poisoning" refers to the inhalation or consumption of lead or lead products into the body even in a minute amount. Lead was used in the paint on walls and other products commonly found in the house. As a result, many people grew up inhaling the chemical and thereby, damaging their health.

Advances in chemistry in these past three decades have dramatically decreased the use of lead in paint. In this way, lead poisoning does not pose the same threat that it did several decades ago. However, the problem still remains acute for families who live in decrepit buildings that have not been repainted since the discovery of the chemical's toxicity. (20. B) Daily inhalation of lead leads to its accumulation in the body. This amount can be considerable, especially for young children whose bodies are smaller and immune systems weaker.

19. What is this talk mainly about?   A)（主旨概括）

20. According to the talk, which one of the following places might be considered dangerous?

                                                         B)（具体细节）

21. Where does the talk most probably take place?   D)（判断推理）

Passage Three (Word count: 191)

The time of the day when something is done can give a special meaning to the event. In the United States, if you telephone someone early in the day, while he is shaving or having breakfast, the time of the call shows that the matter is very important and requires immediate attention. (23. C)

Imagine the excitement and fear caused by a crowd of people arriving at the door at 2:00 a.m. on an island in the South Pacific. A factory manager from the United States has just had such an experience. The natives met one night to discuss a problem. When they arrived at a solution, they went to see the factory manager and woke him up to tell him what had been decided. (24. B) Unfortunately, it was after two o'clock in the morning. They did not know that it is a serious matter to wake up Americans at this hour. The factory manager did not understand the local culture, and he thought there was a fight and he called the police. It never occurred to him that parts of the day have different meanings in different cultures. (22. D)

22. What is the talk mainly about?   D)（主旨概括）

23. What is not an appropriate time to telephone someone for trivial matters?   C)（判断推理）

24. Why did the natives go to the plant manager's house and wake him up?   B)（具体细节）

Passage Four (Word count: 158)

Every day at least eight Americans choke to death. Their deaths occur because choking is often confused with heart attack, or because old remedies are not successful.

However, the Heimlich maneuver, developed in 1947, is an easily-applied technique to help save the choking victim. (25. D) It must be applied quickly, for the choking victim has but four or five minutes to live after an object is stuck in his throat. The technique involves several procedures, depending on whether the victim is standing, sitting, or lying down, but the basic maneuver is the following: Make a fist with your hand, place it on the abdomen above the belly button and below the ribcage, and press in and upward with a quick thrust. (26. C) The procedure may be repeated several times if necessary until enough force is applied to eject the object. If you are alone and choking, you should use your own fist, or press into a table or a sink. (27. B)

25. What is the talk mainly about?   D)（主旨概括）

26. What is the basic manoeuvre of the Heimlich technique?   C)（具体细节）

27. Which of the following statements is true?   B)（判断推理）

Passage Five (Word count: 153)

In the near future, diagnosing a patient illness may become much less painful for the patient and less uncertain for the doctor. Research and technological advances in scientific photography may ultimately enable a doctor to discover a patient's problem with pictures rather than with blood and tissue samples. (28. B) Such new diagnostic techniques may even help doctors detect diseases much earlier than they could using conventional techniques. One new technique is thermography, a photographic process in which variations in temperature within the body show up as different colors. (29. C) Even at rest the temperatures of different areas of the body are constantly changing. This technique of measuring the variations of body temperature graphically has a great advantage over X-rays and other conventional diagnostic methods. With thermography there are no side effects, no uncomfortable exploratory procedures, and there is no need to take blood and tissue samples. Patients need not endure pain or fear unknown procedures. (30. A)

28. What is the main subject of the talk?   B)（主旨概括）

29. How do thermographic pictures indicate the temperatures of various parts of the body?

C)（具体细节）

30. According to the speaker, why will thermography be non-threatening to patients?   A)（判断推理）

* * *

听力成绩分析表

项目名称	正确	错误	原因	备注
对话				
片段				
听力总分				

注：原因可分为①粗心；②走神；③懵了；④根本就听不懂。

Practice Test 2

PAPER ONE

Part I   Listening Comprehension (30%)

Section A

Directions: *In this section, you will hear five conversations. At the end of each conversation, you will hear three questions about the conversation. The question will be spoken only once. After you hear the question, read the four possible answers marked A, B, C, and D. Choose the best answer and mark the letter of your choice on the* **ANSWER SHEET**.

Sample Answer

A B ● D

Listen to the following example.

You will hear:

W: Can you tell me about yourself, please?

M: Sure, my name's Harry, 18 years old, currently studying biology and chemistry at school. As you are aware, I hope to pursue a career in medicine.

W: Harry, why do you want to be a doctor?

M: Well, everyone in my family is a doctor, so I think I can follow on nicely. (2. A)

W: Apart from treating patients, what do you think being a doctor is going to require?

M: Well, you also need to be academic and have to be an excellent communicator (3. B) with your team and the patients.

Question No. 1: What are the two speakers talking about?

You will read:

1.   A. Switching to biology and chemistry.

     B. Choosing to be a family physician.

     C. Going to college.

     D. **Being a doctor.**

The correct answer is D. Mark the right answer on the **ANSWER SHEET** *as indicated below:*

1. A   B   C   ●

Question No. 2: Why does Harry choose to be a doctor?

You will read:

2.   A. **Because of his family influence.**

     B. Because of the fact that he's young.

     C. Because of the practical skills he has.

     D. Because of his love for biology and chemistry.

The correct answer is A. Mark the right answer on the **ANSWER SHEET** *as indicated below:*

2. ●   B   C   D

Question No. 3: What is mentioned by Harry as one of the requirements for a doctor?
You will read:

3. A. A strong sense of responsibility.

    B. **Good communicative skills**.

    C. Excellent health.

    D. Great patience.

The correct answer is B. Mark the right answer on the **ANSWER SHEET** *as indicated below:*

3. A ● C D

Now let's begin with Conversation One.

Conversation One

1. A. Inability to capture idiomatic expressions.   B. Lack of linguistic skills.

    C. Complicated emotions.   D. Inefficient speed.

2. A. Efficiency and speed.

    B. Accurate word-for-word translation.

    C. Understanding nuances and cultural context.

    D. Ability to replace AI systems.

3. A. Replacing human translators with AI systems.

    B. Relying solely on AI systems for translations.

    C. Ignoring the benefits of AI in translation.

    D. Collaborating between human and AI machine translators.

Conversation Two

4. A. How one can become a good negotiator.

    B. Differences between a good negotiator and a poor one.

    C. How to control one's emotions when negotiating.

    D. Ways to succeed in a hard negotiation.

5. A. They know when to stop.

    B. They know how to adapt.

    C. They know when to make compromises.

    D. They know how to control their emotions.

6. A. A good negotiator is always firm and confident.

    B. A good negotiator never compromises.

    C. A poor negotiator's emotion is not stable.

    D. A poor negotiator can also learn fast.

Conversation Three

7. A. The effects of climate change.   B. A Spanish dance festival.

    C. A great love story.   D. A plan for going out.

8. A. She hasn't been out for many years.   B. She likes films about climate change.

    C. She does not like anything depressing.   D. She is not interested in dance.

9. A. At 7:00 P.M.   B. At 7:30 P.M.

    C. At 7:00 A.M.   D. At 7:30 A.M.

Conversation Four

10. A. Most of her schoolmates are younger than she is.

B. She worries she won't fit in as a transfer student.

C. There are too many activities for her to cope with.

D. She simply has no idea what school to transfer to.

11. A. Participate in after-school activities.

B. Pick up some meaningful hobbies.

C. Seek advice from senior students.

D. Look into what the school offers.

12. A. He doesn't understand transfer students.

B. He can't deal with Catherine's problem.

C. He is warm-hearted and helpful.

D. He is reluctant to offer any help.

Conversation Five

13. A. A special gift from the man.   B. A call from the woman's dad.

C. The woman's lucky birthday.   D. The woman's wedding anniversary.

14. A. Gave her a big model plane.   B. Bought her a gold necklace.

C. Took her on a trip overseas.   D. Threw her a surprise party.

15. A. He is eager to learn how the couple's holiday turns out.

B. He wants to find out about the couple's holiday plan.

C. He will be glad to be a guide for the couple's holiday trip.

D. He will tell the woman the secret if her husband agrees.

Section B

Directions: *In this section, you will hear five passages. At the end of each passage, you will hear three questions about the passage. The question will be spoken only once. After you hear the question, read the four possible answers marked A, B, C, and D. Choose the best answer and mark the letter of your choice on the* **ANSWER SHEET**.

Sample Answer

A   B   ●   D

Passage One

16. A. The harms of social media to mental health.

B. The benefits of social media for communication.

C. The role of online communities in mental well-being.

D. The importance of using social media mindfully.

17. A. Increased feelings of happiness and contentment.

B. Enhanced self-esteem and confidence.

C. Increased likelihood of online bullying and harassment.

D. Improved mental well-being and overall health.

18. A. By distorting their sense of reality.

B. By creating a constant need for validation.

C. By causing increased feelings of depression and anxiety.

D. By providing a platform for online support communities.

Passage Two

19. A. Bad effects of chronic lateness.   B. Reasons for chronic lateness.

C. Suggestions for chronic lateness.   D. All of the above.

20. A. It has spoiled friendship and caused the latecomer to lose his or her job.
    B. It caused the latecomer to lose his or her reputation.
    C. It has aroused other people's resentment.
    D. It has helped the latecomer to be distinctive.

21. A. To be patient.   B. To be punctual.
    C. To get an appointment earlier.   D. To be tolerant.

Passage Three

22. A. Poison control centres and doctors.   B. Bathing from a container or in the shower.
    C. Water temperature, as it affects eyeballs. D. First aid treatment of eye problems.

23. A. High fever.
    B. Allergic reactions or inflammations.
    C. The foreign substance can be absorbed through the eye.
    D. Chemical burns.

24. A. Fifteen minutes.   B. Two or three inches.
    C. Immediately.   D. Into the inside corner of the eye.

Passage Four

25. A. How pharmaceutical companies make money from cold drugs.
    B. Common colds and their remedies.
    C. Antibodies are less numerous than folk remedies.
    D. Isolate yourself to avoid cold.

26. A. The common colds are not infectious.
    B. Patients with the common colds cough and sneeze.
    C. Cold viruses can survive for a limited time.
    D. The common colds can spread through physical contact.

27. A. There is an efficient way to prevent it.
    B. People know its cause and how to cure it.
    C. Antibodies quickly produced can counter the effects of viruses.
    D. There are many medicines that can cure it.

Passage Five

28. A. Impaired memory of patients.   B. Cures for Alzheimer's disease.
    C. The use of rats as experimental subjects. D. Nerve growth factor as a cure for Alzheimer's.

29. A. To find a cure for Alzheimer's disease.
    B. To undo the effects of the impaired memory.
    C. To find out an appropriate dose for Alzheimer's.
    D. To test if the deterioration can be stopped.

30. A. Alzheimer's disease is deadly.
    B. Nerve growth factor can reverse the general process of memory deterioration.
    C. The experiments showed some benefits from nerve growth factor.
    D. More work needs to be done to understand the effects of nerve growth factor.

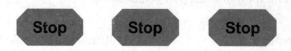

模拟答题卡

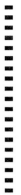

姓　　名	

准考证号	

| 报考学校 | |

| 填涂说明 | 正确填涂 ● 　　错误填涂 ⊘ ⊗ ⊘ ⦶ ⊘ ⊖ |

考生须知

1.答题前，考生务必用黑色字迹签字笔或水笔将姓名、准考证号、报考学校填写清楚。
2.按照题号顺序在各题目的答题区域内作答，未在对应的答题区域作答或超出答题区域的作答均不给分。
3.选择题用2B铅笔作答，不得使用涂改液。

缺考违纪标记栏：　缺考 ○　　作弊 ○　　（此项由监考人员填涂！）

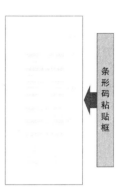

条形码粘贴框

选择题

1	(A)	(B)	(C)	(D)	16	(A)	(B)	(C)	(D)
2	(A)	(B)	(C)	(D)	17	(A)	(B)	(C)	(D)
3	(A)	(B)	(C)	(D)	18	(A)	(B)	(C)	(D)
4	(A)	(B)	(C)	(D)	19	(A)	(B)	(C)	(D)
5	(A)	(B)	(C)	(D)	20	(A)	(B)	(C)	(D)
6	(A)	(B)	(C)	(D)	21	(A)	(B)	(C)	(D)
7	(A)	(B)	(C)	(D)	22	(A)	(B)	(C)	(D)
8	(A)	(B)	(C)	(D)	23	(A)	(B)	(C)	(D)
9	(A)	(B)	(C)	(D)	24	(A)	(B)	(C)	(D)
10	(A)	(B)	(C)	(D)	25	(A)	(B)	(C)	(D)
11	(A)	(B)	(C)	(D)	26	(A)	(B)	(C)	(D)
12	(A)	(B)	(C)	(D)	27	(A)	(B)	(C)	(D)
13	(A)	(B)	(C)	(D)	28	(A)	(B)	(C)	(D)
14	(A)	(B)	(C)	(D)	29	(A)	(B)	(C)	(D)
15	(A)	(B)	(C)	(D)	30	(A)	(B)	(C)	(D)

书面表达　请用黑色签字笔在答题区域内作答，超出边框无效！

Detailed Explanations of Answers to Practice Test 2

Part Ⅰ Listening Comprehension—Tapescript and Answer Keys
Section A
Conversation One (Word count: 109)

W: Hey, have you ever noticed how AI-powered translation systems are posing some challenges?

M: Oh yeah, definitely. They're getting better, but let's be real. They still can't beat human translators.

W: No doubt about that. Machines struggle with the small details, like cultural context and idioms. (1. A)

M: True, humans can really grasp the subtle meanings behind words. (2. C)

W: Absolutely. But, hey, we can't deny that AI has its perks when it comes to efficiency and speed.

M: Yeah, it's got its benefits, but we shouldn't overlook the value of human expertise and language skills.

W: I'm with you on that. Maybe a collaboration between human translators and AI could be the way to go, huh? (3. D)

1. What is a challenge mentioned by the speakers about AI machine translation systems?
    A)（主旨概括）
2. What advantage do human translators have over machines?
    C)（具体细节）
3. How to use AI machine translation systems alongside human translators?
    D)（判断推理）

Conversation Two (Word count: 137)

W: Mr. Green, what do you think makes a successful negotiator? (4. B)

M: Well, that's hard to define. But I think successful negotiators have several things in common. They are always polite and rational people. They are firm but flexible. They can recognize power and how to use it. They are sensitive to the dynamics of the negotiation, the way of rises and falls and how it may change direction. They project the image of confidence, and perhaps most importantly, they know when to stop. (5. A)

W: And, what about an unsuccessful negotiator? (4. B)

M: Well, this is probably all of us when we start out. We are probably immature and over-trusting, too emotional or aggressive. (6. C) We are unsure of ourselves and we want to be liked by everyone. Good negotiators learn fast. Poor negotiators remain like that and go on losing negotiations.

4. What is the conversation mainly about?
    B)（主旨概括）
5. What may be the most important thing to a successful negotiator?
    A)（具体细节）
6. What can be inferred from the conversation?
    C)（判断推理）

Conversation Three (Word count: 136)

M: Do you feel like going out tonight? (7. D)

W: Yeah, why not? We haven't been out for ages! What's on?

M: Well, there is a film about climate change. Does it sound good to you?

W: Oh, not really. It doesn't really appeal to me. What's it about? Just climate change?

M: I think it's about how climate change affects everyday life. I wonder how they make it entertaining.

W: Well, it sounds really awful. It's an important subject, I agree. But I'm not in the mood for anything depressing. (8. C) What else is on?

M: There's a Spanish dance festival.

W: Oh, I love dance. That sounds really interesting.

M: Apparently, it's absolutely brilliant. Let's see what it says in the paper. Anna Gomez leads in an exciting production of a great Spanish love story, Carmen.

W: Okay then, what time is it on?

M: At 7:30. (9. B)

    7. What is the conversation mainly about?   D)（主旨概括）

    8. What do we learn about the woman from the conversation?   C)（判断推理）

    9. When will the Spanish love story be on?   B)（具体细节）

Conversation Four (Word count: 139)

W: Good morning, Mr. Lee, may I have a minute of your time?

M: Sure, Catherine. What can I do for you? (12. C)

W: I'm quite anxious about transferring over to your college. I'm afraid I won't fit in. (10. B)

M: Don't worry, Catherine. (12. C) It's completely normal for you to be nervous about transferring schools. This happens to many transfer students.

W: Yes, I know, but I'm younger than most students in my year and that worries me a lot.

M: Well, you may be the only younger one in your year, but you know we have a lot of afterschool activities you can join in, (11. A) and so this way, you'll be able to meet new friends of different age groups.

W: That's nice! I love games and hobby groups.

M: I'm sure you do. So you will be just fine. (12. C)

W: Thanks so much. I definitely feel better now.

    10. Why does Catherine feel anxious?   B)（主旨概括）

    11. What does the man encourage Catherine to do?   A)（具体细节）

    12. What do we learn about the man?   C)（判断推理）

Conversation Five (Word count: 137)

M: I bet you're looking forward to the end of this month. Are you?

W: Yes, I am. How did you know?

M: David told me you had a special birthday coming up.

W: Oh...yeah that's right. This year will be my golden birthday. (13. C)

M: What does that mean?

W: A golden or lucky birthday is when one turns the age of their birth date. So, for example, my sister's birthday is December 9th and her golden birthday would have been the year she turned nine years old. Come to think of it, my parents did throw her a surprise party that year. (14. D)

M: Interesting. I assume you got big plans then.

W: Actually yes. My husband is planning a surprise trip for the two of us next week.

M: Have a fantastic time. I can't wait to hear all about it when you get back. (15. A)

    13. What are the two speakers talking about?   C)（主旨概括）

    14. What did the woman's parents do on her sister's golden birthday?   D)（具体细节）

    15. What does the man say at the end of the conversation?   A)（判断推理）

Section B

Passage One (Word count: 147)

    Nowadays, social media has become an integral part of our lives. It allows us to connect with friends, share our thoughts, and discover new information. However, there are concerns about the negative impact of excessive social media use on mental health. (16. A)

Several studies have found a link between social media and increased feelings of depression, anxiety, and loneliness. Spending too much time scrolling through social media feeds can lead to a distorted sense of reality and a constant need for validation. Additionally, cyberbullying and online harassment are prevalent issues that can further harm mental well-being. (17. C)

On the positive side, social media also offers opportunities for connection and support. Online communities and support groups can provide a sense of belonging and resources for individuals facing similar challenges. It is important to use social media in a balanced and mindful way, prioritizing mental health and taking breaks when needed. (18. D)

16. What is the main topic of the passage?　　　　　　　　　　　　A)（主旨概括）
17. What are the harmful effects of the overuse of social media?　　　C)（具体细节）
18. How can social media positively impact individuals' mental health?　D)（判断推理）

Passage Two (Word count: 173)

Chronic lateness has spoiled friendships, and it's a habit that has caused people to lose their jobs. (20. A) Why, then, are so many people late?

"Not arriving on time can be a form of avoidance," says Dr. Richard Kronsky, a psychiatrist at Lexington Medical Center in Massachusetts."You're late for a party, or coming home from work, because you don't want to be where you're supposed to be."

Other reasons for chronic lateness are more complicated. Dr. Kronsky suggests that some latecomers know that their lateness will cause anger, and this serves their deep need to be punished. Alternatively, some latecomers have a tendency to force someone to wait, which is a way of expressing anger or resentment.

As for those of us who wait, we can set limits as to how long we will stay before leaving. When appropriate, we can make our anger known. And though it is true that being prompt can be as compulsive as being late, Shakespeare advised this:"Better three hours too soon than a minute too late."(21. C)

19. What is the talk mainly about?　　　　　　　　　　　　　　　D)（主旨概括）
20. What effects created by chronic lateness are mentioned in the passage?　A)（具体细节）
21. What does the passage finally advise us to do?　　　　　　　　　C)（判断推理）

Passage Three (Word count: 149)

Many substances that come into contact with the surface of the eye can cause chemical burns, allergic reactions or inflammations, or even be absorbed through the eye. (23. A) Whenever one of these types of substances does come into contact with someone's eye, the eye should be flushed out immediately with water. Lukewarm water should be poured gently into the inside corner of the eye from a container two or three inches above the victim's eye. (24. B) A water tap will do very nicely as it produces controllable pressure. The victim's head should be tilted so that the water will flow across the eyeball and off the face. This procedure should be followed for five to fifteen minutes, depending on the severity of the problem. Adults who are not otherwise incapacitated may use a shower to wash out the eyes. Urgency is the key word in treating eye problems of this sort.

22. What is the topic of this talk?　　　　　　　　　　　　　　　D)（主旨概括）
23. Which of the following is NOT a result of the eye accident?　　　A)（具体细节）
24. How far from the victim's head should the water be poured?　　　B)（具体细节）

Passage Four (Word count: 157)

Every year millions of us fall victim to the common cold. As the symptoms include coughing and sneezing, it is widely assumed that colds are spread through the air to be inhaled by other sufferers. But research has shown that cold viruses can survive for a limited time on a number of surfaces, including human skin. So they can also be passed on through physical contact. (26. A) The only efficient way to avoid spreading or catching a cold is to isolate yourself completely, though this is hardly practical. Colds are rarely serious as antibodies are quickly produced to counter the effects of the cold-producing virus, which may be any one of hundreds. (27. C) Commercially produced cold cures are many and provide an important source of income for pharmaceutical companies. There are also numerous folk remedies. I prefer to try and drown the cold bugs in alcohol. It may do little for the cold but it certainly cheers me up.

    25. What is the main topic of this talk?   B)（主旨概括）

    26. Which of the following is NOT true?   A)（判断推理）

    27. Why are colds rarely serious?   C)（具体细节）

Passage Five (Word count: 172)

    Alzheimer's disease impairs a person's ability to recall memories, both distant memories and memories as recent as a few hours ago. Although there is not yet a cure for the illness, there may be hope for a cure with a protein called nerve growth factor. Scientists from the University of Lund in Sweden and the University of California at San Diego designed an experiment to test whether doses of nerve growth factor could reverse the effects of memory loss caused by Alzheimer's. (29. B) Using a group of rats with impaired memory, the scientists gave half of the rats doses of nerve growth factor while giving the other half a blood protein as a placebo, thus creating a control group. At the end of the four-week test, the rats given the nerve growth factor performed equally to rats with normal memory abilities. While the experiments do not show that nerve growth factor can stop the general process of deterioration caused by Alzheimer's, they do show potential as a means to slow the process significantly. (30. D)

    28. What is the topic of this passage?   D)（主旨概括）

    29. What was the purpose of the experiment in the passage?   B)（具体细节）

    30. Which of the following can be inferred from the passage?   D)（判断推理）

* * *

听力成绩分析表

项目名称	正确	错误	原因	备注
对话				
片段				
听力总分				

注：原因可分为①粗心；②走神；③懂了；④根本就听不懂。

Practice Test 3

PAPER ONE

Part I   Listening Comprehension (30%)

Section A

Directions: *In this section, you will hear five conversations. At the end of each conversation, you will hear three questions about the conversation. The question will be spoken only once. After you hear the question, read the four possible answers marked A, B, C, and D. Choose the best answer and mark the letter of your choice on the ANSWER SHEET.*

Sample Answer

A B ● D

Listen to the following example.

You will hear:

> W: Can you tell me about yourself, please?
>
> M: Sure, my name's Harry, 18 years old, currently studying biology and chemistry at school. As you are aware, I hope to pursue a career in medicine.
>
> W: Harry, why do you want to be a doctor?
>
> M: Well, everyone in my family is a doctor, so I think I can follow on nicely. (2. A)
>
> W: Apart from treating patients, what do you think being a doctor is going to require?
>
> M: Well, you also need to be academic and have to be an excellent communicator (3. B) with your team and the patients.

Question No. 1: What are the two speakers talking about?

You will read:

1. A. Switching to biology and chemistry.
    B. Choosing to be a family physician.
    C. Going to college.
    D. **Being a doctor.**

The correct answer is D. Mark the right answer on the ANSWER SHEET as indicated below:

1.A   B   C   ●

Question No. 2: Why does Harry choose to be a doctor?

You will read:

2. A. **Because of his family influence.**
    B. Because of the fact that he's young.
    C. Because of the practical skills he has.
    D. Because of his love for biology and chemistry.

The correct answer is A. Mark the right answer on the ANSWER SHEET as indicated below:

2. ●   B   C   D

Question No. 3: What is mentioned by Harry as one of the requirements for a doctor?
You will read:

3. A. A strong sense of responsibility.
    B. **Good communicative skills**.
    C. Excellent health.
    D. Great patience.

The correct answer is B. Mark the right answer on the **ANSWER SHEET** *as indicated below:*

3. A ● C D

Now let's begin with Conversation One.

Conversation One

1. A. Handling a traffic accident.   B. Consulting for an emergent problem.
    C. Making an emergency call.   D. Making an appointment with the doctor.
2. A. His wife has just passed away.   B. His wife has lost consciousness.
    C. He suffers from shortness of breath.   D. He suffers from depression.
3. A. The man's is too anxious to speak clearly.   B. The man has difficulty breathing.
    C. The man's English is foreign-accented.   D. The man has aphasia.

Conversation Two

4. A. Her heavy smoking.   B. Her heavy sputum.
    C. Her worries about work.   D. Her persistent cough.
5. A. Smoking and work.   B. Drinking and family.
    C. Work and family.   D. Smoking and drinking.
6. A. How she lost her job.   B. Her cough and other symptoms.
    C. How she tried to quit smoking.   D. Why she has so many health problems.

Conversation Three

7. A. Insomnia.   B. Dementia.
    C. Autism.   D. Leukeamia.
8. A. He takes it the first thing in the morning.   B. He memorizes it again and again.
    C. He asks others to remind him.   D. He always has a good memory.
9. A. He can name a pencil but can't use it.   B. He can use a pencil but can't name it.
    C. He is more than 88 years old.   D. His wife died a long time ago.

Conversation Four

10. A. She has difficulty with her present job.
    B. She wants to get rid of her chest infection.
    C. The antibiotics doesn't work for her and has some side effects.
    D. She is worried about losing her job.
11. A. Thrush.   B. Exhausted.
    C. Still feeling bad after taking the antibiotics.   D. Insomnia.
12. A. The antibiotics don't fit the patient.   B. The side effect takes time to disappear.
    C. The patient doesn't complete the course.   D. The patient works for too long a time.

Conversation Five

13. A. He might have a stroke.   B. He has a drinking problem.
    C. He might have a heart attack.   D. His blood pressure is slightly high.
14. A. Flushing out extra fluid and salt in the body.

    B. Helping the patient to lose some weight.

    C. Blocking the effects of adrenalin on the heart.

    D. Reducing the amount of stress to the heart.

15. A. Take diuretics.   B. Take beta-blocks.

    C. Give up alcohol soon.   D. Change his life-style.

Section B

Directions: *In this section, you will hear five passages. At the end of each passage, you will hear three questions about the passage. The question will be spoken only once. After you hear the question, read the four possible answers marked A, B, C, and D. Choose the best answer and mark the letter of your choice on the* **ANSWER SHEET.**

Sample Answer

A B ● D

Passage One

16. A. Sleep deficit in the US.   B. How to sleep well.

    C. Facts and myths about sleep.   D. US's insomniac population.

17. A. 35 million.   B. 34 million.

    C. 25 million.   D. 20 million.

18. A. Sleeping in 8-hour consolidated blocks.

    B. Sleeping during the daytime.

    C. Going to bed soon after dark.

    D. Two blocks of 4-hour sleep with a waking break.

Passage Two

19. A. The pitfalls of stress.   B. How to manage stress.

    C. The realities of stress.   D. Why stress is bad.

20. A. It has become widespread.   B. It is not necessary for life.

    C. It has been around since the Garden of Eden.   D. There are both good and bad stresses.

21. A. By finding out how to get rid of it.   B. By exercising vigorously.

    C. By getting more of it.   D. By getting the right amount of it.

Passage Three

22. A. They were always short of time.   B. They were very forgetful.

    C. They were very frightened of flying.   D. They often suffer from airsickness.

23. A. A stamp.   B. An envelope.

    C. Two tickets.   D. Some flight insurance.

24. A. An empty envelope.   B. Some coins.

    C. The insurance policy.   D. The tickets.

Passage Four

25. A. The advantages and disadvantages to contact lenses.

    B. The popularity of contact lenses.

    C. The cost of contact lenses.

    D. The cosmetic benefits of contact lenses.

26. A. They correct vision more effectively.   B. They create natural peripheral vision.

    C. They never steam up.   D. They are less costly.

27. A. $175 to $275.   B. $150 to $250.

    C. $215 to $315.   D. $450 to $600.

Passage Five

28. A. The impact of enzymes on chemical reactions.
    B. The way the body produces enzymes.
    C. The structure of enzymes.
    D. Types of chemical products created with enzymes.

29. A. It divides into two different parts.
    B. It keeps the same chemical structure.
    C. It becomes part of a new chemical compound.
    D. It produces more of the enzyme.

30. A. Energy is needed to start a biochemical reaction with enzymes.
    B. Enzymes can speed up biochemical reactions.
    C. Enzymes work following the principle of efficiency.
    D. Enzymes can lower the number of biochemical reactions.

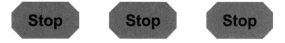

模拟答题卡

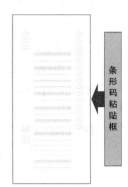

姓　名	
准考证号	
报考学校	

考生须知

1.答题前，考生务必用黑色字迹签字笔或水笔将姓名、准考证号、报考学校填写清楚。
2.按照题号顺序在各题目的答题区域内作答，未在对应的答题区域作答或超出答题区域的作答均不给分。
3.选择题用2B铅笔作答，不得使用涂改液。

填涂说明　正确填涂 ●　错误填涂 ⊘⊗⊙⊖

缺考违纪标记栏：　缺考 ○　　作弊 ○　　（此项由监考人员填涂！）

条形码粘贴框

选择题

1	(A)	(B)	(C)	(D)	16	(A)	(B)	(C)	(D)
2	(A)	(B)	(C)	(D)	17	(A)	(B)	(C)	(D)
3	(A)	(B)	(C)	(D)	18	(A)	(B)	(C)	(D)
4	(A)	(B)	(C)	(D)	19	(A)	(B)	(C)	(D)
5	(A)	(B)	(C)	(D)	20	(A)	(B)	(C)	(D)
6	(A)	(B)	(C)	(D)	21	(A)	(B)	(C)	(D)
7	(A)	(B)	(C)	(D)	22	(A)	(B)	(C)	(D)
8	(A)	(B)	(C)	(D)	23	(A)	(B)	(C)	(D)
9	(A)	(B)	(C)	(D)	24	(A)	(B)	(C)	(D)
10	(A)	(B)	(C)	(D)	25	(A)	(B)	(C)	(D)
11	(A)	(B)	(C)	(D)	26	(A)	(B)	(C)	(D)
12	(A)	(B)	(C)	(D)	27	(A)	(B)	(C)	(D)
13	(A)	(B)	(C)	(D)	28	(A)	(B)	(C)	(D)
14	(A)	(B)	(C)	(D)	29	(A)	(B)	(C)	(D)
15	(A)	(B)	(C)	(D)	30	(A)	(B)	(C)	(D)

书面表达　请用黑色签字笔在答题区域内作答，超出边框无效！

Detailed Explanations of Answers to Practice Test 3

Part Ⅰ　Listening Comprehension—Tapescript and Answer Keys

Section A

Conversation One (Word count: 106)

W: Dr. Thompson's office. How can I help you?

M: I need a doctor right now.

W: Tell me the problem, sir.

M: My wife just passed out. (2. B)

W: Sir, it's difficult to understand you. Please take a deep breath and calm down. (3. A)

M: My wife's just passed out. I am not sure what to do. So I call in.

W: All right, sir. Dr. Thompson is handling an emergency case right now. But he will come to you in 5 minutes.

M: I think my wife is dying. Isn't this an emergency? (1. C)

W: Yes, sir, of course. Please be patient. Here is the doctor.

   1.　What is the conversation concerned about?　　　　　　　　　　C)（主旨概括）

   2.　Why does the man make the call?　　　　　　　　　　　　　B)（具体细节）

   3.　Why does the woman have difficulty understanding the man?　　A)（判断推理）

Conversation Two (Word count: 135)

M: Your doctor says that you have a cough. Could you please tell me more about it and about any other symptoms you may have? (6. B)

W: Well, I've had this cough for about 2 months now and sometimes I feel short of breath, particularly in the morning. (4. D)

M: Could you tell me if you bring up any sputum when you cough?

W: Yes, sometimes I do in the morning but I think that's because I smoke, although I am trying to cut down. Also, I wheeze, particularly when I'm at work and I think that's due to the air conditioning.

M: You seem to have two concerns. First, you want to stop smoking (5. A) and I am sure that this is important for your health. Second, you are worried about your work. (5. A) How do you think that I can help?

   4.　What problem brings the woman to the man?　　　　　　　　D)（主旨概括）

   5.　What are the woman's concerns?　　　　　　　　　　　　　A)（具体细节）

   6.　What does the man want to learn from the woman?　　　　　　B)（判断推理）

Conversation Three (Word count: 122)

W: Do you ever forget to take your medication?

M: No, I never do.

W: How do you remember?

M: That's the first thing I do every day. (8. A) But sometimes my memory is not so good. Sometimes I forget things I'm going to say. (7. B)

W: Is that a new problem for you?

M: No, it has been for some time. I guess at 88. (9. C)

W: At 88 I think you're doing fine. Can I test your memory so we can get an idea of how much of a problem it is?

M: Okay.

W: Please name this for me.

M: Well, I don't know. (7. B)

W: Would you know how to use it?

M: No. I couldn't even write anymore.

W: You know it is for writing?

M: I have no idea. (7. B)

W: Okay, well it's a pencil.

    7. What is the patient's problem?   B)（主旨概括）

    8. How does the patient remember to take his medication?   A)（具体细节）

    9. What do we learn about the patient from the conversation?   C)（判断推理）

Conversation Four (Word count: 92)

M: Hello, Miss Lennox. What can I do for you?

W: The antibiotics you prescribed haven't cleared up my chest infection.

M: Right. Did you complete the course?

W: Yes, I did.

M: And do you feel any better after taking them?

W: Um, no. They've had absolutely no effect, apart from giving me thrush and leaving me feeling completely washed out. (10. C) (11. D)

M: Right. I'm sorry to hear that. Sometimes antibiotics may not agree with patients. (12. A) What I'll do is try you with a different antibiotic and see how that goes.

    10. What's the problem with the patient?   C)（主旨概括）

    11. Which of the following doesn't the patient complain of?   D)（具体细节）

    12. How does the doctor explain the problem?   A)（判断推理）

Conversation Five (Word count: 192)

W: Mm, your blood pressure is a bit on the high side, Mr. Dean. (13. D)

M: Oh.

W: I'll take it again in a few minutes ... It's gone down a little, but it's still a bit higher than it should be. It's important that we control it. Do you understand why it's important to control your blood pressure?

M: It can cause a stroke or heart attack?

W: Yes, that's right. Now, there are a number of options you could consider. So firstly, I'll outline what they are and then I'll talk about each treatment in turn. OK?

M: Fine.

W: In terms of medication, the following options are available. You could consider taking water pills, or diuretics. (15. C) These flush out excess fluid and salt in your body, (14. A) which helps to lower blood pressure.

M: Ah.

W: Another option is taking beta blockers. (15. C) Basically, these block the effects of adrenalin on the heart, reducing the amount of stress to the heart. This means the heart doesn't have to work so hard, and therefore blood pressure is reduced. And the third option you could think about at this stage is making certain adjustments to your current life-style... (15. C)

    13. What's the patient's problem?   D)（主旨概括）

14. What is the effect of diuretics according to the doctor?　　　　　　　　A)（具体细节）

15. Which of the following the doctor DOESN'T advise?　　　　　　　　　　C)（判断推理）

Section B

Passage One (Word count: 151)

Our culture is obsessed with sleep and the lack of it. Yet many of us don't know some basic facts. (16. C) As many as 35 million Americans experience chronic insomnia. (17. A) And yet in 2006, only 20 million dollars were spent on research. Here are five common myths about how we get our shut-eye and why. (16. C)

One, humans need 8 hour-sleep a night. There are many ways of sleeping, and few cultures sleep in 8 hours consolidated blocks like we do. Until the industrial era, many western Europeans divided the night into the first sleep and the second sleep. They go to bed soon after dark, sleep for 4 hours, and then wake for an hour or two during which they write, pray, smoke, have sex, or even visit neighbors. In fact, there are some evidence to suggest that this sleep pattern may be the most in tune with our inherent circadian rhythm. (18. D)

16. What is the conversation mainly about?　　　　　　　　　　　　　　C)（主旨概括）

17. According to the talk, how many Americans suffer from chronic insomnia?　　A)（具体细节）

18. Which sleeping pattern may best fit our inherent biological system?　　　　D)（判断推理）

Passage Two (Word count: 165)

Stress comes in all shapes and sizes, and has become so pervasive, that it seems to permeate everything and everybody. Some doctors refer to stress as some kind of new plague. Why all of the commotion? After all, stress has been around since Adam and Eve were in the Garden of Eden. Stress is an unavoidable consequence of life. (19. C) Without stress, there would be no life. (20. B) However, just as distress can cause disease, there are good stresses that offset this, and promote wellness. Increased stress results in increased productivity—up to a point. However, this level differs for each of us. It's very much like the stress on a violin string. Not enough strain produces a dull, raspy sound. Too much makes a shrill, annoying noise, or causes the string to snap. However, just the right degree can create magnificent tones. Similarly, we all need to find the proper level of stress that promotes optimal performance, and enables us to make melodious music. (21. D)

19. What aspect of stress is the talk mainly about?　　　　　　　　　　C)（主旨概括）

20. What is NOT true about stress?　　　　　　　　　　　　　　　　　B)（具体细节）

21. How can we deal with stress according to the passage?　　　　　　　　D)（判断推理）

Passage Three (Word count: 196)

Let me tell you a story about Bert and Mildred Bumbridge, who used to be very forgetful. (22. B) For example, Mildred would forget to cook dinner, or Bert would show up for work on Sunday thinking it was Monday. One summer they were to take a long plane trip. What do you suppose happened? Well, they got to the airport with only ten minutes to spare. So time was short. In that situation anyone would board the plane right away. But not Mr. and Mrs. Bumbridge. They just had to buy some flight insurance first. After all, who knows what will happen on a plane flight? They quickly put some coins into a machine and out came their insurance policy. (23. D)"Who would get the money if we crash, I wonder?" asked Mildred. "My mother, of course," her husband replied."We'll mail the policy to her. Now quick, give me a stamp, will you?" he said. (24. C)"The plane's going to take off in another minute." Bert put the stamp on the envelope, dropped it in the mail box, and suddenly let out a cry. What happened do you suppose? He had mailed their plane tickets to his mother!

22. What does this passage tell us about Bert and Mildred Bumbridge?　　　B)（主旨概括）

23. What did Bert and Mildred get after putting coins into the machine?　　　D)（具体细节）

24. What did Bert want to mail to his mother? C)（具体细节）

Passage Four (Word count: 150)

There are several advantages to contact lenses. (25. A) The contact lenses correct vision more effectively than eyeglasses. Since they move with your eye, you can always see through the lens's optical center. The result is crisp images, excellent depth perception, and natural peripheral vision. Contact lenses also have cosmetic benefits. They never steam up or get rain-splattered, and they never slip down your nose.

On the other hand, contact lenses are costly. (26. D) You'll probably spend a few hundred dollars a year on the chemical cleaning system alone. Disposable contacts cost even more. (27. C) There are two types of conventional contact lenses: soft lens and rigid gas-permeable lens. Soft lenses cost about $175 to $275 for the original fitting. Rigid gas-permeable lenses cost about $25 more. The cost for disposable contacts is between $450 to $600 for a year's supply. (27. C) And unfortunately, there is some degree of eye infections and eye diseases with contacts.

25. What is the talk mainly about? A)（主旨概括）

26. Which of the following is NOT mentioned as an advantage of contact lenses? D)（具体细节）

27. Which of the following is likely to be the yearly cost of rigid gas-permeable lenses? C)（判断推理）

Passage Five (Word count: 147)

Let's begin today by discussing enzymes. Enzymes are what make many of the body's biochemical reactions possible. (28. A) Actually, biochemical reactions can take place without them, but at much lower rates. In fact, an enzyme may cause a reaction to proceed billions of times faster than it would otherwise. (29. B)

There are two reasons that enzymes are so effective at enabling biochemical reactions. First, enzymes greatly reduce the amount of energy required to start the reactions, and with much less energy needed, the reactions can proceed a lot faster than they could without the enzyme. (30. D) The second reason is that only a small amount of an enzyme is needed to enable the biochemical reaction. That's because the chemical structure of the enzyme itself does not become altered as it enables the reaction. (29. B) So a single enzyme can be used to start the same biochemical reaction over and over again.

28. What is the talk mainly about? A)（主旨概括）

29. What point does the professor make about an enzyme when it is involved in a biochemical reaction?

B)（具体细节）

30. Which is NOT true according to the passage? D)（判断推理）

* * *

听力成绩分析表

项目名称	正确	错误	原因	备注
对话				
片段				
听力总分				

注：原因可分为①粗心；②走神；③懵了；④根本就听不懂。

Practice Test 4

PAPER ONE

Part I Listening Comprehension (30%)

Section A

Directions: *In this section, you will hear five conversations. At the end of each conversation, you will hear three questions about the conversation. The question will be spoken only once. After you hear the question, read the four possible answers marked A, B, C, and D. Choose the best answer and mark the letter of your choice on the* **ANSWER SHEET**.

Sample Answer

A B ● D

Listen to the following example.

You will hear:

    W: Can you tell me about yourself, please?

    M: Sure, my name's Harry, 18 years old, currently studying biology and chemistry at school. As you are aware, I hope to pursue a career in medicine.

    W: Harry, why do you want to be a doctor?

    M: Well, everyone in my family is a doctor, so I think I can follow on nicely. (2. A)

    W: Apart from treating patients, what do you think being a doctor is going to require?

    M: Well, you also need to be academic and have to be an excellent communicator .(3. B) with your team and the patients.

Question No. 1: What are the two speakers talking about?

You will read:

1.   A. Switching to biology and chemistry.

     B. Choosing to be a family physician.

     C. Going to college.

     D. **Being a doctor.**

The correct answer is D. Mark the right answer on the **ANSWER SHEET** *as indicated below:*

1. A B C ●

Question No. 2: Why does Harry choose to be a doctor?

You will read:

2.   A. **Because of his family influence.**

     B. Because of the fact that he's young.

     C. Because of the practical skills he has.

     D. Because of his love for biology and chemistry.

The correct answer is A. Mark the right answer on the **ANSWER SHEET** *as indicated below:*

2. ● B C D

Question No. 3: What is mentioned by Harry as one of the requirements for a doctor?
   You will read:

3.   A. A strong sense of responsibility.

   B. **Good communicative skills**.

   C. Excellent health.

   D. Great patience.

   The correct answer is B. Mark the right answer on the **ANSWER SHEET** *as indicated below:*

                                             3. A ● C D

Now let's begin with Conversation One.

Conversation One

1.   A. The man's travel to Portland.   B. The man's headache.
   C. The man's symptoms.   D. The man's breathing difficulty.

2.   A. A difficult case.   B. A trivial illness.
   C. A deadly disease.   D. A serious condition.

3.   A. Cough.   B. Fever.
   C. Stuffed nose.   D. Sore throat.

Conversation Two

4.   A. Her face-cream.   B. Her smelly face-cream.
   C. Her skin rash.   D. Side effects of her medication.

5.   A. She began to use an expensive face cream since her birthday.

   B. She has been on some anti-oxidation medication.

   C. She is allergic to nice-smelling ice-cream.

   D. She broke up with her boy-friend on her birthday.

6.   A. The Chinese face-cream.   B. The American face-cream.
   C. The French perfume.   D. The medication.

Conversation Three

7.   A. The woman's ECG.   B. The woman's test results.
   C. The woman's blood pressure.   D. The woman's stomach upsets.

8.   A. White blood cell count.   B. Red blood cell count.
   C. X-ray.   D. ECG.

9.   A. Too much work to do.   B. A heavy load of studying.
   C. Her daughter's sickness.   D. Her insufficient income.

Conversation Four

10. A. Swine Flu.   B. Coronavirus pneumonia.
   C. Bird Flu.   D. Bronchitis.

11. A. It is a genetic disorder.   B. It is a respiratory condition in pigs.
   C. It is an illness from birds to humans. D. It is a gastric ailment.

12. A. Eating pork.   B. Eating chicken.
   C. Raising pigs.   D. Breeding birds.

Conversation Five

13. A. Giving a vaccine injection to the woman.   B. Preparing for an intravenous injection.
   C. Drawing blood for a sample test.   D. Giving a bleeding therapy.

14. A. To warn her of the danger.   B. To persuade to give up the test.

C. To distract her attention.   D. To comfort and calm her.

15. A. The woman's condition is critical.
    B. The woman has been picking up quite well.
    C. The woman's illness was caused by a mosquito bite.
    D. The woman won't see the doctor any more.

Section B

Directions: *In this section, you will hear five passages. At the end of each passage, you will hear three questions about the passage. The question will be spoken only once. After you hear the question, read the four possible answers marked A, B, C, and D. Choose the best answer and mark the letter of your choice on the* **ANSWER SHEET.**

Sample Answer
A B ● D

Passage One

16. A. A multipurpose AI language model that generates human-like text responses.
    B. An advanced chat platform for social interactions.
    C. An OpenAI project aimed at understanding human language patterns.
    D. An algorithm that collects and analyzes Internet text data.

17. A. Limited functionality and narrow task support.
    B. Inability to interact through voice assistants.
    C. Ability to answer questions and provide recommendations.
    D. Strict reliance on context and nuanced queries.

18. A. Constant incorrect and incoherent answers.
    B. Inability to understand complex queries and ambiguity.
    C. Consistently producing human-like responses.
    D. Revolutionizing technology interaction.

Passage Two

19. A. The decline of authentic human connections.
    B. The secure use of personal information.
    C. The potential spread of misinformation.
    D. The improvement of AI chatbots' performance.

20. A. The ethical use of AI capabilities.
    B. The potential decline in authentic human connections.
    C. The optimization of AI chatbot performance.
    D. The improvement of social and psychological consequences.

21. A. Unauthorized access to user conversations.
    B. The generation of biased or offensive responses.
    C. The ethical implementation of AI chatbots.
    D. The spread of misinformation.

Passage Three

22. A. Smoking and lung cancer.   B. Lung cancer and the sexes.
    C. How to quit smoking.   D. How to prevent lung cancer.

23. A. Current smokers exclusively.   B. Second-hand smokers.
    C. With a lung problem.   D. At age 40 or over.

24. A. 156.   B. 269.
    C. 7,498.   D. 9,427.

Passage Four

25. A. A hobby.   B. The whole world.
    C. A learning experience.   D. A career to earn a living.

26. A. Her cervical vertebrae were seriously injured.
    B. Her shoulders were severely injured.
    C. Her arms were broken.
    D. Her legs were broken.

27. A. She learned a foreign language.   B. She learned to make friends.
    C. She learned to be a teacher.   D. She learned living skills.

Passage Five

28. A. Life evolution.   B. Space exploration.
    C. Extraterrestrial life.   D. Unknown flying objects.

29. A. His 50th birthday.
    B. NASA's 50th anniversary.
    C. The University's 50th anniversary.
    D. The US Cosmology Association's 50th anniversary.

30. A. Even primitive life is impossible.   B. Intelligent life is fairly common.
    C. Intelligent life is less likely.   D. Any form of life is possible.

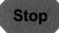 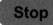

模拟答题卡

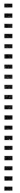
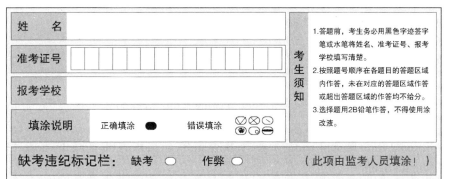
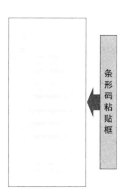

选择题	1	(A)	(B)	(C)	(D)	16	(A)	(B)	(C)	(D)
	2	(A)	(B)	(C)	(D)	17	(A)	(B)	(C)	(D)
	3	(A)	(B)	(C)	(D)	18	(A)	(B)	(C)	(D)
	4	(A)	(B)	(C)	(D)	19	(A)	(B)	(C)	(D)
	5	(A)	(B)	(C)	(D)	20	(A)	(B)	(C)	(D)
	6	(A)	(B)	(C)	(D)	21	(A)	(B)	(C)	(D)
	7	(A)	(B)	(C)	(D)	22	(A)	(B)	(C)	(D)
	8	(A)	(B)	(C)	(D)	23	(A)	(B)	(C)	(D)
	9	(A)	(B)	(C)	(D)	24	(A)	(B)	(C)	(D)
	10	(A)	(B)	(C)	(D)	25	(A)	(B)	(C)	(D)
	11	(A)	(B)	(C)	(D)	26	(A)	(B)	(C)	(D)
	12	(A)	(B)	(C)	(D)	27	(A)	(B)	(C)	(D)
	13	(A)	(B)	(C)	(D)	28	(A)	(B)	(C)	(D)
	14	(A)	(B)	(C)	(D)	29	(A)	(B)	(C)	(D)
	15	(A)	(B)	(C)	(D)	30	(A)	(B)	(C)	(D)

书面表达 请用黑色签字笔在答题区域内作答,超出边框无效!

_____

_____

_____

Detailed Explanations of Answers to Practice Test 4

Part Ⅰ　Listening Comprehension—Tapescript and Answer Keys

Section A

Conversation One (Word count: 142)

W: Oh? Are you feeling bad?

M: I have been sick for a week and I am scheduled to fly to Portland this weekend.

W: What sort of symptoms?

M: Mostly are sinus infection. I can't breathe and I've got yellow stuffs and I keep blowing my nose. (3. C)

W: How is it with your mouth open?

M: That's fine. But I can't go around like some kind of fish, you know?

W: Okay, then, stuffy head, nasal drainage. What else?

M: That's it. That's enough. (2. B) Usually I get these colds and they go on one or two days. This time I had all week.

W: I see, and any other symptoms? Cough, fever, anything else?

M: No. Maybe a tick in my throat. I cough once or twice, no big deal though. (2. B)

W: Ok, let's take a look at you.

　1.　What are the man and woman talking about?　　　　　　　　　　　C)（主旨概括）

　2.　How would you describe the man's illness?　　　　　　　　　　　B)（具体细节）

　3.　What is the worst symptom of the man?　　　　　　　　　　　　C)（判断推理）

Conversation Two (Word count: 100)

W: My skin has suddenly gone rough and red, and spots keep breaking out. Is there anything that I can do?

M: Have you used anything different on your face? Have you been on any medication?

W: I usually use this Chinese face-cream. But on my birthday I got some very expensive American face-cream which smelled very nice. I wonder if that could be the problem. (5. A)

M: Do you have the face cream with you?

W: Yes, here it is.

M: It smells very strong. Maybe you are allergic to the perfume in it. (6. B) I suggest you stop using it immediately.

　4.　What problem brings the woman to the man?　　　　　　　　　　C)（主旨概括）

　5.　Which of the following is true about the woman?　　　　　　　　A)（具体细节）

　6.　What might be the cause for the woman's problem?　　　　　　　B)（判断推理）

Conversation Three (Word count: 136)

M: Well, your ECG is perfectly normal, and there is no problem with your X-ray, either. But your white blood cell count is rather high, (8. A) which is what I expected as it shows your body is fighting the virus. (7. B)

W: Is there anything you can give me to make me feel better, doctor? I am very busy at work this week, and I have a lot of studying to do. But I don't feel up for it. Also my daughter is still in bed and... (9. D)

M: Don't worry, it's just gastric flu, but I will give you some medicine for it to make you feel better. Three times a day take the white tablets as directed on the label after meal. And for the charcoal tablets, take one or two depending on how loose your bowels are.

7. What is the topic of the conversation? B）（主旨概括）

8. According to the woman's test result, which of the following items is abnormal? A）（具体细节）

9. Which of the following is NOT a reason for the woman's anxiety? D）（具体细节）

Conversation Four (Word count: 180)

W: Hello, Doctor Smith. Could you tell us something about swine flu?

M: Well, it's a common respiratory ailment in pigs that doesn't usually spread to people. (11. B)

W: But why are so many people infected?

M: Unlike most cases, this flu virus appears to be a subtype not seen before in humans or pigs. It has genetic material from pigs, birds and humans, according to the WHO.

W: Then why is it called swine flu? Were pigs the carriers of this virus?

M: Hmm. It's closer to say that pigs were the mixing ball for this virus.

W: What does that mean?

M: I mean, birds can't pass bird flu to people. But pigs are susceptible to getting flu viruses that infected birds. The viruses inside the infected pig might mutate in form that could also infect other mammals.

W: Wow, so complicated. By the way, can we catch swine flu from eating pork?

M: Actually, ill pigs are not allowed to enter the market. Cooking also kills the virus. Only people who work with pigs can catch the virus. (12. C)

10. What are the speakers talking about? A）（主旨概括）

11. What do we know about the disease? B）（具体细节）

12. What may cause people to have swine flu? C）（判断推理）

Conversation Five (Word count: 90)

W: What might be wrong with me, doctor?

M: Mm. I don't know at the moment. But I will take some blood sample from you for a lab exam. (13. C) Is that all right?

W: Sure, doctor.

M: Well, just keep your arms straight there. Fine, there will be a little prick, like a mosquito bite. (14. D) OK? There we go, OK. I will send that sample off and we'll check it. (13. C) If the sample is OK, we won't need to go on seeing you any more.

W: So you think I'm getting better?

M: Absolutely. (15. B)

13. What is the man doing according to the conversation? C）（主旨概括）

14. Why does the man tell the woman that "there will be a little prick like mosquito bite"?

D）（具体细节）

15. What can be inferred from the conversation? B）（判断推理）

Section B

Passage One (Word count: 162)

ChatGPT is an advanced AI language model developed by OpenAI. It is designed to generate human-like text responses and engage in conversational interactions. (16. A) ChatGPT uses a deep learning algorithm that trains on vast amounts of text data from the Internet, allowing it to understand and generate coherent responses.

One of the key advantages of ChatGPT is its versatility. It can provide help with various tasks, such as answering questions, providing recommendations (17.C) or even engaging in casual conversations. Users can interact with ChatGPT through different platforms, including websites, messaging apps, and voice assistants.

However, it is important to note that ChatGPT has limitations. It can sometimes produce incorrect or nonsensical answers, as it relies solely on the information it has been trained on. Additionally, ChatGPT may not understand complex or nuanced queries and may struggle with context or ambiguity. (18. B)

Overall, ChatGPT represents a significant advancement in AI language models and has the potential to revolutionize how we interact with technology and access information.

16. What is ChatGPT and what is its main function?   A)（主旨概括）

17. What are some advantages of using ChatGPT?   C)（具体细节）

18. What are some limitations of ChatGPT?   B)（具体细节）

Passage Two (Word count: 141)

As ChatGPT gains popularity, some people have expressed concerns about its potential implications. One worry is the ethical use of AI and the possible misuse of ChatGPT's capabilities. There are concerns about the spread of misinformation or the generation of harmful content, (19. C) as ChatGPT can inadvertently produce biased or offensive responses.

Another worry is the impact on human interaction. Critics argue that increased reliance on AI chatbots like ChatGPT may lead to a decline in authentic human connections. (20. B) They fear that individuals may become reliant on machines for social interactions, which could have profound social and psychological consequences.

Lastly, there are concerns about privacy. AI chatbots gather vast amounts of user data to improve their performance, raising questions about the security and protection of personal information. (21. A) Data breaches or unauthorized access to user conversations are significant worries in this context.

While ChatGPT offers numerous benefits, addressing these worries is crucial for its responsible and ethical implementation.

19. What is one of the worries associated with ChatGPT?   C)（主旨概括）

20. What are critics concerned about regarding the rising dependence on AI chatbots?   B)（具体细节）

21. What privacy concern is associated with AI chatbots like ChatGPT?   A)（判断推理）

Passage Three (Word count: 150)

For years, researchers have debated whether smoking affects the lungs of men and women differently. And in the most compelling studies on the topic to date, researchers are determined that women are twice vulnerable to lung cancer as men. But in a surprising twist, they die at half the rate of men. The study, which was published last week in the Journal of American Medical Association, included 9,427 men and 7,498 women from throughout north America who were healthy, at least 40 years old, (23. D) and in the range of former smokers. Over the course of more than eight years, a group of investigators led by Doctor Claudia Hemshky of the Wile Medical College of New York City identified lung tumours in 113 of the men and 156 of the women. (24. B) Then the researchers kept track of who lived and for how long as well as the treatment the participants were given.

22. What is the talk mainly about?   A)（主旨概括）

23. What was one of the requirements to the participants of the study?   D)（具体细节）

24. Over the course of more than 8 years, how many of the participants developed lung cancer?

B)（具体细节）

Passage Four (Word count: 155)

Joe was an average skier, competing and winning numerous titles in junior and senior national ski events. As Joe says, "Skiing was it, everything, my world." (25. B) Joe's world collapsed on January 30th, 1955 when she skied off the outer round and landed helplessly on the slope. Her fourth, fifth and sixth cervical vertebrae were broken. (26. A) For days, Joe hovered between life and death. By April it became clear that she would be paralyzed from the shoulders down. Joe underwent rehabilitation therapy with cheerful determination. She learned to write, to type and to feed herself. Once she had mastered daily living skills, she enrolled in a university in California at Los Angeles, where she studied art, German and English. (27. D) After overcoming yet another personal tragedy, the death of her boyfriend in a plane crash, Joe graduated in 1961. By this time, Joe had chosen a new career goal, teaching elementary school children.

25. What did ski mean to Joe before the accident?　　　　　　　　　　　　B)（具体细节）

26. What happened to Joe when she skied off the outer round?　　　　　　　A)（具体细节）

27. What did Joe learn during her rehabilitation?　　　　　　　　　　　　D)（具体细节）

Passage Five (Word count: 170)

Steven Hawking: Life on other planets is likely, (28. C) but intelligent life is less likely. Famed astrophysicist Stephen Hawking has been thinking a lot about the cosmic question, "Are we alone?" The answer is probably not, he says. If there is life elsewhere in the universe, Hawking asks why we haven't stumbled onto some alien broadcasts in space, maybe something like "alien quiz shows". Hawking's comments were part of the lecture at George Washington University on Monday in honour of NASA's 50th anniversary. (29. B) He theorized that there are possible answers to whether there is extraterrestrial ET life. One option is that there likely isn't any life elsewhere. Or maybe there is intelligent life elsewhere, but it gets smart enough to send signals into space; it is also smart enough to make destructive nuclear weapons（核武器）. Hawking said he prefers the third opinion: "Primitive life is very common and intelligent life is fairly rare," (30. C) he then quickly added: "Some would say it has yet to occur on earth."

28. What is the passage mainly about?　　　　　　　　　　　　　　　　　C)（主旨概括）

29. What is the event when Hawking delivered his lecture at George Washington University?

　　　　　　　　　　　　　　　　　　　　　　　　　　　　　　　　　B)（具体细节）

30. What is the idea Hawking favours in terms of extraterrestrial life?　　　　C)（具体细节）

* * *

听力成绩分析表

项目名称	正确	错误	原因	备注
对话				
片段				
听力总分				

注：原因可分为①粗心；②走神；③懵了；④根本就听不懂。

Practice Test 5

PAPER ONE

Part I Listening Comprehension (30%)

Section A

Directions: *In this section, you will hear five conversations. At the end of each conversation, you will hear three questions about the conversation. The question will be spoken only once. After you hear the question, read the four possible answers marked A, B, C, and D. Choose the best answer and mark the letter of your choice on the **ANSWER SHEET**.*

Sample Answer
A B ● D

Listen to the following example.

You will hear:

W: Can you tell me about yourself, please?

M: Sure, my name's Harry, 18 years old, currently studying biology and chemistry at school. As you are aware, I hope to pursue a career in medicine.

W: Harry, why do you want to be a doctor?

M: Well, everyone in my family is a doctor, so I think I can follow on nicely. (2. A)

W: Apart from treating patients, what do you think being a doctor is going to require?

M: Well, you also need to be academic and have to be an excellent communicator (3. B) with your team and the patients.

Question No. 1: What are the two speakers talking about?

You will read:

1.   A. Switching to biology and chemistry.
     B. Choosing to be a family physician.
     C. Going to college.
     D. **Being a doctor.**

*The correct answer is D. Mark the right answer on the **ANSWER SHEET** as indicated below:*

1. A B C ●

Question No. 2: Why does Harry choose to be a doctor?

You will read:

2.   A. **Because of his family influence.**
     B. Because of the fact that he's young.
     C. Because of the practical skills he has.
     D. Because of his love for biology and chemistry.

*The correct answer is A. Mark the right answer on the **ANSWER SHEET** as indicated below:*

2. ● B C D

Question No. 3: What is mentioned by Harry as one of the requirements for a doctor?
You will read:

3.   A. A strong sense of responsibility.
     B. **Good communicative skills**.
     C. Excellent health.
     D. Great patience.

The correct answer is B. Mark the right answer on the **ANSWER SHEET** *as indicated below:*

3. A ● C D

Now let's begin with Conversation One.

Conversation One

1.   A. Mr. Peters' family medical history.
     B. Mr. Peters' health checkup status.
     C. Mr. Peters' past medical history.
     D. Mr. Peters' memory problem.

2.   A. Amnesia.   B. Hypertension.
     C. Ischemia.   D. Minor stroke.

3.   A. His problem may be related to his family medical history.
     B. His uncle's bad health made him frustrated.
     C. Irregular pulse runs in his family.
     D. Strokes bothered him a lot.

Conversation Two

4.   A. Achievement of Martin.   B. Personality of Martin.
     C. Martin's performance on the project.   D. Martin's difficulty in the project.

5.   A. She can't do the presentation.   B. She's not sure what the assignment is.
     C. She doesn't understand the theory.   D. She has problems applying the theory.

6.   A. He knows the project thoroughly.
     B. He knew much from the beginning to the end.
     C. He is quiet at the beginning of the year.
     D. He has problems with his assignment.

Conversation Three

7.   A. The uniqueness of King Salmon.   B. The glacier water of the Copper River.
     C. Linda's brother.   D. A dinner cooked by Sarah.

8.   A. Sarah and Brian.   B. Brian and Linda.
     C. Linda and her brother.   D. The woman and her friend.

9.   A. The King River in Alaska.   B. The Copper River in Alaska.
     C. Prince William Sound.   D. The Alaska River.

Conversation Four

10. A. How to stretch.   B. How to change ideas.
     C. How to pull a tooth.   D. How to exhale.

11. A. In a doctor's office.   B. In an exercise class.
     C. In a dentist's office.   D. In a biology class.

12. A. Gaining new concepts.   B. Releasing stress.
     C. Stretching.   D. Pulling teeth.

Conversation Five

13. A. The patient is calling the doctor's office to make an appointment.
    B. The man is calling to book a ticket.
    C. The man is calling to make a reservation.
    D. The receptionist is making a phone call.

14. A. To cash a check.   B. To check up on the work.
    C. To change the appointment.   D. To have a physical checkup.

15. A. Miss Ortega is the doctor to whom the man is making an appointment.
    B. This is the first time Bill Jackson to see the doctor.
    C. Bill Jackson is not urgent to see the doctor.
    D. The doctor is free for the next few weeks.

Section B

Directions: *In this section, you will hear five passages. At the end of each passage, you will hear three questions about the passage. The question will be spoken only once. After you hear the question, read the four possible answers marked A, B, C, and D. Choose the best answer and mark the letter of your choice on the* **ANSWER SHEET.**

Sample Answer
A B ● D

Passage One

16. A. To tell an anecdote about an author and a baby.
    B. To introduce an author of detective stories.
    C. To tell a miracle of a baby.
    D. To describe a tough disease.

17. A. She was a British girl whose parents were working in Qatar.
    B. The hospitals in Qatar were full at this time.
    C. She was the daughter of a doctor in one of the places.
    D. The Qatar doctors were not sure they could cure her.

18. A. Contact with a pair of infected spectacles.
    B. Contact with a harmful substance used to kill insects.
    C. Contact with machinery used in manufacturing optical glass.
    D. Contact with an adult who carried thallium germs in his body.

Passage Two

19. A. To teach important safety rules.   B. To explain the grading procedures.
    C. To demonstrate an experiment.   D. To tell students what safety equipment to buy.

20. A. Professor Smith.   B. A teaching assistant.
    C. A specialist in chemistry.   D. A university technician.

21. A. Every day of the week.   B. One day a week.
    C. Two days a week.   D. Once every two weeks.

Passage Three

22. A. A Lucky Escape.   B. Mr. Tan's Bravery.
    C. The Work of the Welfare Department.   D. A Terrible Storm.

23. A. 14.   B. 7.
    C. 21.   D. 15.

24. A. It happened early last Friday morning. B. It lasted for more than one hour.
    C. It tore through the New Territories. D. It caused serious damage to the people.

Passage Four

25. A. Predators in the animal world. B. Divisions of the food chain.
    C. The loss of potential energy in predators. D. A parasitic chain.

26. A. A bird eating a fish. B. A rabbit eating grass.
    C. A tapeworm living in an animal. D. A plant using energy from the sun.

27. A. 10 percent. B. 12-15 percent.
    C. 2-3 percent. D. More than 15 percent.

Passage Five

28. A. Ultraviolet light. B. The use of spray cans.
    C. Air-conditioning systems. D. Fluorocarbons and the ozone layer.

29. A. A chemist. B. A professor.
    C. A mechanic. D. A doctor.

30. A. Providing fluorocarbons. B. Shielding the sun.
    C. Protecting the earth. D. Destroying chemicals.

Stop　Stop　Stop

模拟答题卡

姓　　名	
准考证号	
报考学校	

填涂说明　正确填涂 ●　错误填涂 ⊘ ⊗ ◎ ⊕ ⊙ ⊖

缺考违纪标记栏：　缺考 ○　　作弊 ○　　（此项由监考人员填涂！）

考生须知

1.答题前，考生务必用黑色字迹签字笔或水笔将姓名、准考证号、报考学校填写清楚。

2.按照题号顺序在各题目的答题区域内作答，未在对应的答题区域作答或超出答题区域的作答均不给分。

3.选择题用2B铅笔作答，不得使用涂改液。

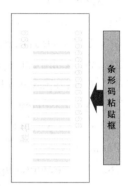

条形码粘贴框

选择题

1	(A)	(B)	(C)	(D)	16	(A)	(B)	(C)	(D)
2	(A)	(B)	(C)	(D)	17	(A)	(B)	(C)	(D)
3	(A)	(B)	(C)	(D)	18	(A)	(B)	(C)	(D)
4	(A)	(B)	(C)	(D)	19	(A)	(B)	(C)	(D)
5	(A)	(B)	(C)	(D)	20	(A)	(B)	(C)	(D)
6	(A)	(B)	(C)	(D)	21	(A)	(B)	(C)	(D)
7	(A)	(B)	(C)	(D)	22	(A)	(B)	(C)	(D)
8	(A)	(B)	(C)	(D)	23	(A)	(B)	(C)	(D)
9	(A)	(B)	(C)	(D)	24	(A)	(B)	(C)	(D)
10	(A)	(B)	(C)	(D)	25	(A)	(B)	(C)	(D)
11	(A)	(B)	(C)	(D)	26	(A)	(B)	(C)	(D)
12	(A)	(B)	(C)	(D)	27	(A)	(B)	(C)	(D)
13	(A)	(B)	(C)	(D)	28	(A)	(B)	(C)	(D)
14	(A)	(B)	(C)	(D)	29	(A)	(B)	(C)	(D)
15	(A)	(B)	(C)	(D)	30	(A)	(B)	(C)	(D)

书面表达　请用黑色签字笔在答题区域内作答,超出边框无效!

Detailed Explanations of Answers to Practice Test 5

Part Ⅰ　Listening Comprehension—Tapescript and Answer Keys

Section A

Conversation One (Word count: 96)

DR: Would you hold out your wrist, please? Let's see ... well, your pulse is regular.

MR. PETERS: Thank you.

DR: Now for your blood pressure ... just fix this around you here, like that ... now, then ...

MR. PETERS: Is it normal?

DR: No, it isn't. Your blood pressure is quite high. (2. B)

MR. PETERS: Really?

DR: Yes. Is there anyone in your family with high blood pressure that you know of?

MR PETERS: My uncle has had it for years. (3. A) I don't recall that it bothered him much, although he did have a stroke a few years ago. That won't happen to me, will it?

DR: No.

1.　What are the two speakers talking about?　　　　　　　　C)（主旨概括）
2.　What is the problem with Mr. Peters?　　　　　　　　　　B)（具体细节）
3.　What can be inferred about Mr. Peters?　　　　　　　　　A)（判断推理）

Conversation Two (Word count: 112)

M: I'm really having trouble with this assignment. How are you doing with it?

W: I'm OK with the theoretical part, but I'm having problems with the application part. (5. D) I'm on my way to ask Martin about it. He knows this project backwards and forwards. Do you want to come with me?

M: Yeah, maybe I will. Martin sure seems to understand things thoroughly.

W: I have to confess something, though. I didn't think he knew much at the beginning of this semester.

M: Yeah. I know what you mean. He's so quiet that at first you don't realize how much he knows. (6. C)

W: Yeah. It takes a while to realize it.

4.　What are the two speakers talking about?　　　　　　　　C)（主旨概括）
5.　What is the woman's difficulty with the assignment?　　　　D)（具体细节）
6.　What can we know from the conversation about Martin?　　　C)（具体细节）

Conversation Three (Word count: 129)

M: Hi Sarah, where are you hurrying off to?

W: Oh hi, Brian. I'm headed over to Linda's house. Her brother just flew in from Alaska with some King Salmon. They're cooking a big dinner. (8. C) Do you like salmon?

M: Yes, I like all kinds of fish, but I've never tasted King Salmon from Alaska. What's so special about it?

W: Well, for one thing, it has a very short season; it's only about a month long each year.

M: So what else makes this King Salmon so special?

W: Well, this fish comes from the glacier water of the Copper River that flows into Prince William Sound in Alaska, (9. B) and this river is really long and fast moving. So the King Salmon have to adapt to that environment.

7. What are the two speakers talking about? A)（主旨概括）

8. Who of the following are probably cooking the dinner? C)（判断推理）

9. Where does King Salmon come from? B)（具体细节）

Conversation Four (Word count: 135)

W: In today's class, (10.A) I want to discuss and demonstrate one of the principles of relaxation exercise. (11. B) This might be different from other ways you've been taught to exercise. What I want you to do is this: stretch your body to the point where you feel a little pull. (10. A) Then stop stretching, but keep the same posture and exhale deeply. By doing this, you will allow your body to release the stress and reduce the resistance. Then you will be able to stretch further, relax, and have no pain.

M: But Susan, I've been doing exercises for years, and for me it always hurts to stretch. (12. C) And sometimes I feel that the pain is good. In fact, if I don't feel the pain, I think that maybe I'm not stretching enough. You know the old saying, "No pain, no gain!"

10. What does this woman mainly want to explain? A)（主旨概括）

11. Where does this conversation probably take place? B)（判断推理）

12. According to the man, what is painful? C)（具体细节）

Conversation Five (Word count: 132)

W: Good afternoon, Dr. Parker's office. Can you hold a second?

M: Uh, yes, sure. (*Pause for a few seconds*.)

W: Thank you for waiting. This is Miss Ortega speaking. Can I help you?

M: My name is Bill Jackson. I would like to make an appointment with Dr. Parker. (13. A)

W: Have you been here to see Dr. Parker before?

M: Yes. I'm one of his regular patients.

W: Is it urgent or can it wait?

M: No, it's not urgent. No emergency. (15. C)

W: We're filled up for the next few weeks.

M: I just want to get a checkup. (14. D)

13. What is going on in this talk? A)（主旨概括）

14. What does the man want to do with the doctor? D)（具体细节）

15. Which of the following statements is true according to the conversation? C)（判断推理）

Section B

Passage One (Word count: 196)

In 1977, a dead author of detective stories saved the life of a 19-month-old baby in a most unusual way. The author was Agatha Christie, a gentle married lady and one of the most successful writers of detective stories in the world.

In June 1977, a baby girl became seriously ill in Qatar, near Saudi Arabia. Doctors were unable to diagnose the cause of her illness with confidence, so she was flown to London and admitted to Hammersmith Hospital. (17. D) While doctors were discussing the baby's case, a nurse asked to speak to them.

"Excuse me," said Nurse Marsha Maitland, "but I think the baby is suffering from thallium poisoning."

"What makes you think that?" Dr. Brown said. "Thallium poisoning is extremely rare."

"A few days ago, I was reading a novel called *A Pale Horse* by Agatha Christie," Nurse Maitland explained. "In this book, somebody uses thallium poison, and all the symptoms are described. They're exactly the same as the baby's."

Finally, tests showed that the baby had indeed been poisoned by thallium, a rare metallic substance used in making optical glass. Enquiries revealed that the poison might have come from an insecticide used in Qatar. (18. B)

16. What is the purpose of the author for writing this passage?   A)（主旨概括）

17. Why was the baby sent to London?   D)（具体细节）

18. According to the passage, what caused the baby's illness?   B)（判断推理）

Passage Two (Word count:159)

Hi. My name is John. I'm your teaching assistant for Chemistry l, Professor Smith's class. (20. B) Let me explain a little about this lab section. It's a required meeting, twice a week. (21. C) I expect you to do all the experiments and keep the results in your lab notebook. I'll collect the notebooks every two weeks. You'll be graded on your lab notebooks, your attendance, and quizzes. But the most important information I want to give you today is about the safety procedures. (19. A)

First of all, you must wear shoes that cover your feet in the lab. That means you can't wear thongs or sandals. Tennis shoes are OK. Also, don't wear clothes that have loose baggy parts, like long scarves and necklaces or loose belts. They could get caught in something or fall into a liquid. Another important safety precaution is cleaning up. Be sure to put the waste in the correct containers. We can't mix liquid with paper.

19. What is the main purpose of the talk?   A)（主旨概括）

20. Who is the speaker of this talk?   B)（具体细节）

21. How often does this class meet?   C)（具体细节）

Passage Three (Word count: 151)

Last Friday a storm tore through two villages in the New Territories destroying fourteen homes. (23. A; 24. C) Seven others were so badly damaged that the owners had to leave them, and fifteen others had broken windows or torn roofs. One person was killed, several were badly injured and taken to the hospital, and a number of other people received smaller injuries. Altogether over two hundred people were homeless as a result of the storm.

A farmer, Mr. C. Y. Tan, said that the storm began early in the morning and lasted for over an hour. "I was in the kitchen with my wife and children," he said, "when we heard a loud noise. A few minutes later our house fell down on top of us. We managed to climb out but then I saw one of my children was missing. I went back inside and found him, safe but very frightened."

22. Which of the following would be the best title for the talk?   D)（主旨概括）

23. How many houses were destroyed by the storm?   A)（具体细节）

24. What is NOT true about the storm?   C)（判断推理）

Passage Four (Word count: 170)

I just want to introduce the next area we'll cover: the food chain. Food chains are divided into three types. (25. B) The first one is the predator chain, in which larger animals feed on smaller animals, such as when a bird eats a fish. (26. A) The second is the parasite chain, in which smaller animals live off larger animals, such as a tapeworm living in a cat's intestines. And the third type is the saprophytic chain in which a microorganism feeds off dead matter.

In each type of chain, potential energy is lost at each level. Let's take the example of a green plant. It gets energy from the sun by photosynthesis, but can use only about 2 or 3 percent of the energy that falls on it. (27. C) The plant is then eaten by a rabbit, but the rabbit can use only about 10 percent of the potential energy of the plant. The rabbit is then eaten by a fox, which can use about 12-15 percent of the energy from the rabbit.

25. What is the major topic of this lecture?   B)（主旨概括）

26. Which of the following is an example of a predator chain?   A）（具体细节）

27. How much of the potential energy from the sun can a plant use?   C）（具体细节）

Passage Five (Word count: 168)

Today I'd like to begin a discussion on the problem of the heating up of the earth. First, we'll touch on the relationship between fluorocarbons and the ozone layer. You probably remember that the ozone layer is the protective shield around the earth. It is important to all life because it filters out harmful ultraviolet light from the sun. (30. C) Ozone itself, a form of oxygen, is regularly made by the action of the sun in the upper atmosphere. It is also regularly destroyed by natural chemical processes. The problem now is that too much of the ozone layer is being destroyed. Scientists suspect that certain chemicals, such as fluorocarbons, are contributing to this depletion of the ozone layer. And why is there an increasing number of fluorocarbons in our air? Because we are using more in the manufacturing of common products, such as spray cans, automobile cooling systems, and refrigerators. The chemical pollution from these fluorocarbons can account for some of the ozone losses that have been reported.

28. What is probably the topic of the talk?   D）（主旨概括）

29. Who is most likely the speaker?   B）（判断推理）

30. What is the most important purpose of the ozone layer?   C）（具体细节）

＊＊＊

听力成绩分析表

项目名称	正确	错误	原因	备注
对话				
片段				
听力总分				

注：原因可分为①粗心；②走神；③懵了；④根本就听不懂。

Practice Test 6

PAPER ONE

Part I   Listening Comprehension (30%)

Section A

Directions: *In this section, you will hear five conversations. At the end of each conversation, you will hear three questions about the conversation. The question will be spoken only once. After you hear the question, read the four possible answers marked A, B, C, and D. Choose the best answer and mark the letter of your choice on the* **ANSWER SHEET**.

Sample Answer

A   B   ●   D

Listen to the following example.

You will hear:

W: Can you tell me about yourself, please?

M: Sure, my name's Harry, 18 years old, currently studying biology and chemistry at school. As you are aware, I hope to pursue a career in medicine.

W: Harry, why do you want to be a doctor?

M: Well, everyone in my family is a doctor, so I think I can follow on nicely. (2. A)

W: Apart from treating patients, what do you think being a doctor is going to require?

M: Well, you also need to be academic and have to be an excellent communicator (3. B) with your team and the patients.

Question No. 1: What are the two speakers talking about?

You will read:

1.   A. Switching to biology and chemistry.
      B. Choosing to be a family physician.
      C. Going to college.
      D. **Being a doctor.**

The correct answer is D. Mark the right answer on the **ANSWER SHEET** *as indicated below:*

1. A   B   C   ●

Question No. 2: Why does Harry choose to be a doctor?

You will read:

2.   A. **Because of his family influence.**
      B. Because of the fact that he's young.
      C. Because of the practical skills he has.
      D. Because of his love for biology and chemistry.

The correct answer is A. Mark the right answer on the **ANSWER SHEET** *as indicated below:*

2. ●   B   C   D

Question No. 3: What is mentioned by Harry as one of the requirements for a doctor?
You will read:

3. A. A strong sense of responsibility.
    B. **Good communicative skills**.
    C. Excellent health.
    D. Great patience.

The correct answer is B. Mark the right answer on the **ANSWER SHEET** *as indicated below:*

3. A ● C D

Now let's begin with Conversation One.
Conversation One

1. A. Chest pain and dizziness.
    B. Hot flashes, difficulty sleeping, and mood swings.
    C. Jaw pain and headaches.
    D. Nausea and vomiting.
2. A. Increased flow and longer duration.
    B. Pale color and lightheadedness.
    C. Regular cycles with severe cramps.
    D. Irregular periods and skipped cycles.
3. A. Pain in her lower back.
    B. Dizziness and fainting episodes.
    C. Vaginal dryness and discomfort during sex.
    D. Shortness of breath and chest tightness.

Conversation Two

4. A. The man's suffering from a cold.
    C. The man's fatigue and rundown.
    B. The man's wife's case history.
    D. The man's pneumonia.
5. A. A couple of days.
    C. Six months.
    B. Four years.
    D. Two weeks.
6. A. His wife has seen the doctor before.
    C. His wife persuaded him to see a doctor.
    B. His wife had a minor operation last year.
    D. Two months ago he was at home with a cold.

Conversation Three

7. A. Causes of tooth decay.
    C. A new way to remove tooth decay.
    B. Methods of preventing gum disease.
    D. A pump that delivers a salty-acid solution.
8. A. A pain in the man's tooth.
    C. A talk with the dentist.
    B. An article the man reads.
    D. An appointment the woman has.
9. A. "Painless" means using novocaine to deaden the nerve.
    B. "Painless" is in fact not completely painless.
    C. The man also once had a cavity.
    D. The new method delivers an acid solution to the cavity.

Conversation Four

10. A. Taking a blood test.
    C. Providing medical advice.
    B. Making a private conversation.
    D. Judging the patient's medical condition.
11. A. Malnutrition.
    C. Hypoglycemia.
    B. Hypohemia.
    D. Pneumonia.

12. A. Too few red cells in the blood.　　B. Too few white cells in the blood.
　　C. Lack of vitamin.　　D. Deficient in iron and protein.

Conversation Five

13. A. Places the woman has visited.　　B. A paper the woman is writing for a class.
　　C. School activities they enjoy.　　D. The woman's plans for the summer.

14. A. She takes great interest in visiting historical sites.
　　B. She will visit historical places this summer.
　　C. Her parents like taking children out.
　　D. She never goes out even she grows older.

15. A. To give them lessons on history.　　B. To help them remember their history lessons.
　　C. To relax them during the summer.　　D. To help them writer papers about history.

Section B

Directions: *In this section, you will hear five passages. At the end of each passage, you will hear three questions about the passage. The question will be spoken only once. After you hear the question, read the four possible answers marked A, B, C, and D. Choose the best answer and mark the letter of your choice on the* **ANSWER SHEET.**

Sample Answer

A　B　● 　D

Passage One

16. A. An accident involving a tractor.　　B. A microsurgery to save a baby's arm.
　　C. A 22-month-old baby.　　D. The future of a baby's arm.

17. A. More than ten hours.　　B. Ten hours.
　　C. More than nine hours.　　D. Nine hours.

18. A. A baby was undergoing microsurgery last night to sew back his left arm.
　　B. The two broken parts were packed in ice for the journey to the hospital.
　　C. The doctor assured the mother of 100 percent recovery of the baby's arm.
　　D. The baby's mother was extremely grateful to the doctors.

Passage Two

19. A. Who learn the best from their mistakes.
　　B. Why different age-groups learn differently.
　　C. How fMRI is applied to the research.
　　D. Why children's brain functions differently from the adults'.

20. A. The use of fMRI.　　B. The use of computer tasks.
　　C. The three-way division of the subjects.　　D. The instructions given to the subjects.

21. A. 12-year-olds respond strongly to negative feedback.
　　B. 12-year-olds' brain function the same as 8-year-olds'.
　　C. 8-year-olds' brain function almost the same as adults'.
　　D. 12-year-olds' brain function almost the same as adults'.

Passage Three

22. A. A new concept of diabetes.
　　B. The definition of type 1 and type 2 diabetes.
　　C. The new management of diabetics in the hospital.
　　D. The new development of non-perishable insulin pills.

23. A. Because it vaporizes easily.

    B. Because it becomes overactive easily.

    C. Because it is usually in injection form.

    D. Because it is not stable above 40 degrees Fahrenheit.

24. A. The diabetics can be cured without taking synthetic insulin any longer.

    B. The findings provide insight into how insulin works.

    C. Insulin can be more stable than it is now.

    D. Insulin can be produced naturally.

Passage Four

25. A. Vegetative patients are more aware than they seem.

    B. Vegetative patients retain some control of their eye movements.

    C. EEG scanners may help us communicate with the vegetative patients.

    D. We usually communicate with the brain-dead people by brain-wave scanners.

26. A. The left-hand side of the brain.   B. The right-hand side of the brain.

    C. The central part of the brain.   D. The front part of the brain.

27. A. Lancet.   B. The Brain.

    C. Economist.   D. JAMA.

Passage Five

28. A. Causes of women's greater longevity than men.

    B. Impact of estrogen on women's longevity.

    C. Relation between menstruation and health.

    D. Causes of cardiovascular diseases for women.

29. A. He is a man who has a gene of longevity.   B. He is a professor at Boston University.

    C. He is the owner of the website Time.com.   D. He is the creator of a website on longevity.

30. A. Women don't like red meat as much as men.

    B. The high estrogen level in women makes the difference.

    C. Women develop cardiovascular disease much later than men.

    D. The incidence of cardiovascular disease is much lower in women.

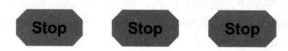

模拟答题卡

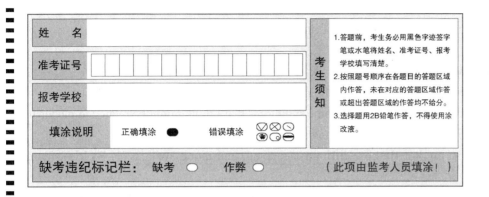

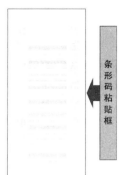

	1	(A)	(B)	(C)	(D)	16	(A)	(B)	(C)	(D)
	2	(A)	(B)	(C)	(D)	17	(A)	(B)	(C)	(D)
	3	(A)	(B)	(C)	(D)	18	(A)	(B)	(C)	(D)
	4	(A)	(B)	(C)	(D)	19	(A)	(B)	(C)	(D)
	5	(A)	(B)	(C)	(D)	20	(A)	(B)	(C)	(D)
	6	(A)	(B)	(C)	(D)	21	(A)	(B)	(C)	(D)
	7	(A)	(B)	(C)	(D)	22	(A)	(B)	(C)	(D)
选	8	(A)	(B)	(C)	(D)	23	(A)	(B)	(C)	(D)
择	9	(A)	(B)	(C)	(D)	24	(A)	(B)	(C)	(D)
题	10	(A)	(B)	(C)	(D)	25	(A)	(B)	(C)	(D)
	11	(A)	(B)	(C)	(D)	26	(A)	(B)	(C)	(D)
	12	(A)	(B)	(C)	(D)	27	(A)	(B)	(C)	(D)
	13	(A)	(B)	(C)	(D)	28	(A)	(B)	(C)	(D)
	14	(A)	(B)	(C)	(D)	29	(A)	(B)	(C)	(D)
	15	(A)	(B)	(C)	(D)	30	(A)	(B)	(C)	(D)

书面表达 请用黑色签字笔在答题区域内作答，超出边框无效！

Detailed Explanations of Answers to Practice Test 6

Part I Listening Comprehension—Tapescript and Answer Keys

Section A

Conversation One (Word count: 120)

M: Hi, Mrs. Johnson. How have you been feeling lately?

W: Hi, doctor. Well, I've been experiencing some symptoms that I think might be related to menopause.

M: I see. Could you please describe the symptoms you've been having?

W: Sure. I've been having hot flashes, difficulty sleeping, and mood swings. (1. B) It's been quite bothersome.

M: Alright. Those symptoms do align with menopausal syndrome. Now, have you noticed any changes in your menstrual cycle?

W: Yes, my periods have become irregular, and sometimes I skip them altogether. (2. D) It's been uncomfortable.

M: Alright. Lastly, have you noticed any issues with vaginal dryness or discomfort during intercourse?

W: Yes, I have experienced some discomfort and dryness. (3. C) It's been uncomfortable.

M: Thank you for sharing that information, Mrs. Johnson. Now, let's discuss the treatment options for managing your symptoms.

    1. What symptoms does the woman experience?   B)（具体细节）

    2. What changes has the woman noticed in her menstrual cycle?   D)（判断推理）

    3. What issue has the woman experienced about her sexual health?   C)（主旨概括）

Conversation Two (Word count: 111)

M: Dr. Brook, I just don't know what's wrong with me. I always feel tired and rundown. (4. C) My wife finally persuaded me to visit you to find out what the trouble is. (6. C)

W: Looking at your case history I see you had pneumonia four years ago and that you also had a minor operation last year. Did you have any long-term aftereffects?

M: Well, I don't remember so...

W: For instance, how long did you stay at home each time?

M: Just a couple of days. (5. A) But about six months ago I was home for about two weeks with a cold or something.

    4. What's the main idea of the conversation?   C)（主旨概括）

    5. How long did the man stay home each time he feels sick?   A)（具体细节）

    6. What is true about the man according to the conversation?   C)（具体细节）

Conversation Three (Word count: 118)

M: Maria, you are leaving early today.

W: Yes, I have a dentist's appointment. (8. D) I put it off as long as I could. But I know I've got at least one cavity.

M: I understand how you feel. I always felt the same until the last time I went to the dentist. (9. C)

W: What changed your mind then?

M: My dentist is using a new method to clean out cavities, and it's painless. (7. C)

W: Painless? You mean after you have a shot of novocaine to deaden the nerve?

M: No, I mean completely painless. The new method uses a pump that delivers a salty-acid solution to the cavity in a pulsating stream.

7. What is the main topic of the talk?   C)（主旨概括）

8. What caused the discussion?   D)（具体细节）

9. Which of the following is true according to the conversation?   C)（具体细节）

Conversation Four (Word count: 72)

M: Blood tests show you are iron deficient. Does that sound right, Mrs. Wilson?

W: I suppose I must be, yes.

M: Now, I want to ask you a few questions to have a clearer idea of <u>what has caused your anaemia. (11. B)</u> I have to ask you a few personal questions if you don't mind. Do you mind if I take a few notes as well as we go along?

W: No, that's fine.

10. What is the conversation mainly about?   D)（主旨概括）

11. What is the patient's problem?   B)（具体细节）

12. Which of the following may be related to the patient's problem?   A)（判断推理）

Conversation Five (Word count: 94)

M: Hi, Janet, you are so lucky to be done with your final exams and term papers. I still have two more finals to take.

W: Really?

M: Yeah. <u>So what are you doing this summer, anything special? (13. D)</u>

W: Well, actually yeah. My parents have always liked taking my sister and me to different places in the United States. <u>You know, places with historical significance. (14. B)</u> <u>I guess they wanted to reinforce the stuff we learned in school about history. And so even though we are older now, they still do once in a while. (15. B)</u>

13. What are these two speakers mainly discussing?   D)（主旨概括）

14. What is true about the woman according to the conversation?   B)（判断推理）

15. Why did the woman's parents take her sister and her to various places?   B)（具体细节）

Section B

Passage One (Word count: 156)

Twenty-two-month-old Ryan Millard of Dalton, Texas, was rushed 100 miles to Las Vegas's Cummington Medical Center after the accident near his home. <u>It took more than ten hours for five surgeons, working through the night, to sew back Ryan Millard's left arm. (17. A)</u>

After Ryan's arm had been broken into two parts, they were packed in ice for the journey to Cummington. Ice keeps a broken limb usable for valuable hours longer so that surgeons have a chance to sew it back.

<u>Now that Ryan has gone through all this, what are his chances of making a complete recovery? About 60 to 40 percent, the doctors said. (18. C)</u>

Hospital secretary, Mr. David Astley, said yesterday, "The operation was technically successful, but it will be some months before we know whether the baby will have 100 percent use of his arm."

Ryan's mother, Mrs. Glynis Millard, said, "We are so grateful to the doctors who have performed this miracle."

16. What is the talk mainly about?   B)（主旨概括）

17. How long did the operation last?   A)（具体细节）

18. Which of the following is NOT true according to the talk?   C)（判断推理）

Passage Two (Word count: 147)

8-year-old children have a radically different learning strategy from 12 year-olds and adults. Eight year-olds learned primarily from positive feedback whereas negative feedback scarcely causes any alarm bells to ring. 12-year-olds are better able to process negative feedback and use it to learn from their mistakes. Adults do the same, but more efficiently. Dr. Eveline Crone and her colleagues from the Leiden Brain and Cognition Lab used fMRI research to compare the brains of three different age groups: (19. A) children of 8 to 9 years, children of 11 to 12 years, and adults aged between 18 and 25 years. This three-way division had never been made before. (20. C) The comparison is generally made between children and adults. Crone herself was surprised by the outcome. We had expected that the brains of 8-year-olds would function exactly in the same way as the brains of 12-year-olds, but maybe not quite as well. (21. B)

19. What is the passage mainly about?　　　　　　　　　　　　　　A)（主旨概括）

20. What is new about Dr. Crone's research?　　　　　　　　　　　C)（判断推理）

21. What had Dr. Crone and her colleagues expected?　　　　　　　B)（具体细节）

Passage Three (Word count: 150)

A team of Australian chemistry students have strengthened the chemical bonds of insulin to make it stable even at room temperatures, a breakthrough that can simplify diabetes management. The findings could shed light on how insulin works, and eventually lead to insulin pills rather than injections or pumps. Insulin needs to be kept cold because it is made of weak chemical bonds that degrade at temperatures above 40 degrees Fahrenheit, making it inactive. (23. D) But using a series of chemical reactions, the research team, comprised of students from Monash University in Australia, replaced the unstable bonds with stronger carbon-based ones. The stronger bonds stabilize the insulins to protein chains without interfering with its natural activity. According to the story about the findings, at Saigru. The so-called diacarbon insulins were stable at room temperatures for several years, Saigru says. Even more promising is that the findings provide an insight into how insulin works. (24. B)

22. What is the main idea of the talk?　　　　　　　　　　　　　D)（主旨概括）

23. Why does the insulin need to be kept cold according to the talk?　　D)（具体细节）

24. What makes the research more promising?　　　　　　　　　　B)（判断推理）

Passage Four (Word count: 156)

Brain-wave scanners might make it possible to communicate with people who are considered brain-dead (25. C), according to a new study reported in the Economist. (27. C) A couple of recent studies have shown that a small minority of vegetative patients (植物人) might be more aware that they seem. Now, Damien Cruse with the medical research council's cognition in brain science unit in Cambridge, UK, thinks, EEG machines will be able to help these patients communicate. The team asked six healthy volunteers to wear EEG devices which connect electrodes to a person's head. They were asked to respond to an audible tone by imagining that they are squeezing their right hands or wiggling the toes of both feet. The researchers found that the volunteers' brain responses were clearly different. The hand squeezing activated the left-hand side of the brain, and toe wiggling produced response in the center of the brain. (26. A)

25. What does this talk mainly tell us?　　　　　　　　　　　　C)（主旨概括）

26. For the six healthy volunteers, which part of the brain did the hand squeezing imagination activate?

A)（具体细节）

27. Where was the study published?　　　　　　　　　　　　　C)（判断推理）

Passage Five (Word count: 164)

Across the industrialized world, women still live 5 to 10 years longer than men. (28. A) Among people over 100 years old, 85% are women, according to Tom Pearls, <u>founder of the New England Centenarian Study at Boston University and creator of the website LivingTo100.com.</u> (29. D) Time.com asks him why. <u>One important reason women live longer than man is the big delay—and advantage women have over men—in terms of cardiovascular disease, like heart attack and stroke.</u> (30. C) Women develop these problems usually in their 70s and 80s, about 10 years later than men. For a long time, doctors thought the difference was due to estrogen. But studies have shown that this may not be the case, and now we know that giving estrogen to women post-menopause can actually be bad for them.

One reason for that delay in onset of cardiovascular disease could be that women are relatively iron-deficient compared to men — especially younger women, those in their late teens and early 20s — because of menstruation.

28. What is the passage mainly about?　　　　　　　　　　　　　　　　　A)（主旨概括）

29. What is true about Tom Pearls, founder of the New England Centenarian Study?　　D)（具体细节）

30. Why do women live longer than men according to Tom Pearls?　　　　　　　C)（判断推理）

* * *

听力成绩分析表

项目名称	正确	错误	原因	备注
对话				
片段				
听力总分				

注：原因可分为①粗心；②走神；③懵了；④根本就听不懂。

Practice Test 7

PAPER ONE

Part I   Listening Comprehension (30%)

Section A

Directions: *In this section, you will hear five conversations. At the end of each conversation, you will hear three questions about the conversation. The question will be spoken only once. After you hear the question, read the four possible answers marked A, B, C, and D. Choose the best answer and mark the letter of your choice on the* **ANSWER SHEET**.

Sample Answer
A B ● D

Listen to the following example.

You will hear:

W: Can you tell me about yourself, please?

M: Sure, my name's Harry, 18 years old, currently studying biology and chemistry at school. As you are aware, I hope to pursue a career in medicine.

W: Harry, why do you want to be a doctor?

M: Well, everyone in my family is a doctor, so I think I can follow on nicely. (2. A)

W: Apart from treating patients, what do you think being a doctor is going to require?

M: Well, you also need to be academic and have to be an excellent communicator (3. B) with your team and the patients.

Question No. 1: What are the two speakers talking about?

You will read:

1.   A. Switching to biology and chemistry.

    B. Choosing to be a family physician.

    C. Going to college.

    D. Being a doctor.

The correct answer is D. Mark the right answer on the **ANSWER SHEET** *as indicated below:*

1. A   B   C   ●

Question No. 2: Why does Harry choose to be a doctor?

You will read:

2.   A. **Because of his family influence.**

    B. Because of the fact that he's young.

    C. Because of the practical skills he has.

    D. Because of his love for biology and chemistry.

The correct answer is A. Mark the right answer on the **ANSWER SHEET** *as indicated below:*

2. ●   B   C   D

Question No. 3: What is mentioned by Harry as one of the requirements for a doctor?
You will read:

3. A. A strong sense of responsibility.
    B. **Good communicative skills**.
    C. Excellent health.
    D. Great patience.

The correct answer is B. Mark the right answer on the **ANSWER SHEET** *as indicated below:*

3. A ● C D

Now let's begin with Conversation One.

Conversation One

1. A. AI's impact on the doctor-patient relationship.
    B. The increasing use of AI in healthcare.
    C. Concerns about patients relying too heavily on AI for diagnoses.
    D. The importance of ensuring AI's complemental role in healthcare.

2. A. Trust-building.   B. Professional opinions.
    C. Empathy and emotional understanding.   D. AI system complexity.

3. A. AI systems might not be cost-effective for healthcare facilities.
    B. Complex AI systems may make patients feel scared or stressed.
    C. AI could potentially replace the need for medical professionals.
    D. Using AI might hinder the trust between doctors and patients.

Conversation Two

4. A. The woman's toothache.   B. Teeth made of plastics.
    C. Tooth transplant.   D. The refill of a tooth.

5. A. The woman prefers filling the bad tooth to taking it out.
    B. They both hate to have a tooth filled.
    C. They both would rather have a tooth filled.
    D. The man prefers to have the bad tooth filled rather than pulled.

6. A. It might grow as a healthy tooth.   B. It might be filled again.
    C. It might get decayed.   D. It might be pulled out.

Conversation Three

7. A. The most absent-minded person.   B. The man's fishing experience.
    C. The man's forgetfulness.   D. The love story between the two speakers.

8. A. On his face.   B. In the bathroom.
    C. The woman had them.   D. Above the mirror.

9. A. His fishing pole.   B. His pants.
    C. His wallet.   D. His boat.

Conversation Four

10. A. The patient's wife's concern for her husband. B. The doctor's worry for the patient.
    C. The patient's suffering from illnesses.   D. The patient's despair of his condition.

11. A. Insomnia.   B. Arthritis.
    C. Nausea.   D. Headaches.

12. A. His arthritis and headaches act up at the same time.
    B. He will quit his job because of bad health.

C. He feels like vomiting because of the headaches.

D. His pain tortured him all day and all night.

Conversation Five

13. A. Two different types of bones in the human body.

 B. How bones help the body move.

 C. How bones continuously repair themselves.

 D. The chemical composition of human bones.

14. A. They were dead.   B. Many things happened in them.

 C. They were dynamic.   D. They repaired themselves.

15. A. Boring.   B. Fascinating.

 C. Useful.   D. Time-consuming.

Section B

Directions: *In this section, you will hear five passages. At the end of each passage, you will hear three questions about the passage. The question will be spoken only once. After you hear the question, read the four possible answers marked A, B, C, and D. Choose the best answer and mark the letter of your choice on the* **ANSWER SHEET.**

Sample Answer

A B ● D

Passage One

16. A. Food Additives.   B. Cancer-related Food.

 C. Food-related Diseases.   D. Bad Effects of Food on Health.

17. A. It has made many additives.   B. It has caused most cancers.

 C. It has made many foods unfit to eat.   D. It makes some cultures more prone to cancer.

18. A. Because of the diet that is characteristic of these cultures.

 B. Because of their living environment.

 C. Because the people of that culture eat much fat.

 D. Because the people of that culture use nitrate and nitrite to preserve color in meats.

Passage Two

19. A. The link between weight loss and sleep deprivation.

 B. The link between weight gain and sleep deprivation.

 C. The link between weight loss and physical exercise.

 D. The link between weight gain and physical exercise.

20. A. More than 68,000.   B. More than 60,800.

 C. More than 60,080.   D. More than 60,008.

21. A. Seven-hour sleepers gained more weight over time than 5-hour ones.

 B. Five-hour sleepers gained more weight over time than 7-hour ones.

 C. Short-sleepers were 15% more likely to become obese.

 D. Short-sleepers consumed fewer calories than long-sleepers.

Passage Three

22. A. Juvenile delinquency.   B. Adolescent mental health.

 C. Adolescent physical problems.   D. Teenage rebellion.

23. A. Combine antidepressants with talk therapy.   B. Promote the transmission between neurons.

 C. Win parental assistance and support.   D. Administer effective antidepressants.

24. A. Family conflicts.   B. Interpersonal conflicts.

     C. Emotion change.   D. Academic pressure.

Passage Four

25. A. Helplessness and worthlessness.   B. Feeling like a loser.

     C. Suicidal feeling.   D. All of the above.

26. A. It encourages the patient to be a top student at school.

     B. It motivates the patient to work better than others.

     C. It makes it easy for the patient to make friends.

     D. It helps the patient hold a positive attitude.

27. A. By encouraging the patient to do the opposite at school.

     B. By urging the patient to face any challenge in reality.

     C. By making the patient aware of his or her existence.

     D. By changing the patient's perspective.

Passage Five

28. A. They sell things at lower prices.   B. They sell different types of small things.

     C. They now sell a lot of hot foods too. D. They are usually of small size.

29. A. They save time and money.   B. They sell better quality merchandise.

     C. They are time-saving and convenient. D. They are impersonal.

30. A. Vending machines are welcomed by customers.

     B. Customers benefit greatly from the creation of vending machines.

     C. Customers usually care a lot about quick service.

     D. Vending machines should not really sell food, cold or hot.

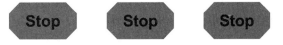

模拟答题卡

姓　　名		
准考证号		
报考学校		
填涂说明	正确填涂　●	错误填涂　⊘⊗⊖⊕⊙⊝

缺考违纪标记栏：　缺考 ○　　作弊 ○　　　　（此项由监考人员填涂！）

考生须知

1.答题前，考生务必用黑色字迹签字笔或水笔将姓名、准考证号、报考学校填写清楚。
2.按照题号顺序在各题目的答题区域内作答，未在对应的答题区域作答或超出答题区域的作答均不给分。
3.选择题用2B铅笔作答，不得使用涂改液。

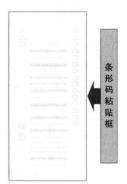

条形码粘贴框

选择题

1	(A)	(B)	(C)	(D)	16	(A)	(B)	(C)	(D)
2	(A)	(B)	(C)	(D)	17	(A)	(B)	(C)	(D)
3	(A)	(B)	(C)	(D)	18	(A)	(B)	(C)	(D)
4	(A)	(B)	(C)	(D)	19	(A)	(B)	(C)	(D)
5	(A)	(B)	(C)	(D)	20	(A)	(B)	(C)	(D)
6	(A)	(B)	(C)	(D)	21	(A)	(B)	(C)	(D)
7	(A)	(B)	(C)	(D)	22	(A)	(B)	(C)	(D)
8	(A)	(B)	(C)	(D)	23	(A)	(B)	(C)	(D)
9	(A)	(B)	(C)	(D)	24	(A)	(B)	(C)	(D)
10	(A)	(B)	(C)	(D)	25	(A)	(B)	(C)	(D)
11	(A)	(B)	(C)	(D)	26	(A)	(B)	(C)	(D)
12	(A)	(B)	(C)	(D)	27	(A)	(B)	(C)	(D)
13	(A)	(B)	(C)	(D)	28	(A)	(B)	(C)	(D)
14	(A)	(B)	(C)	(D)	29	(A)	(B)	(C)	(D)
15	(A)	(B)	(C)	(D)	30	(A)	(B)	(C)	(D)

书面表达　请用黑色签字笔在答题区域内作答，超出边框无效！

Detailed Explanations of Answers to Practice Test 7

Part Ⅰ　Listening Comprehension—Tapescript and Answer Keys

Section A

Conversation One (Word count: 125)

M: You know, the use of AI in healthcare is becoming more widespread, but it's also bringing some challenges to the doctor-patient relationship. (1. A)

W: Oh really? What kind of challenges are you talking about?

M: Well, one concern is that patients might start relying too heavily on AI for diagnoses and not seek professional opinions as often. (1. A)

W: Ah, I see. That could really undermine the trust and connection we establish with our patients.

M: Exactly. On top of that, AI doesn't have empathy or the ability to understand emotional needs like we do. (2. C)

W: That's true. Patients might also feel intimidated or overwhelmed by the complexity of AI systems. (3. B)

M: Absolutely. So, it's important that we make sure AI complements our expertise and improves patient care instead of replacing it.

  1.　What is the main topic of this conversation?　　　　　　　　　A)（主旨概括）

  2.　What aspect of patient care is AI lacking, according to the conversation?　　C)（具体细节）

  3.　What is one potential drawback of heavy dependence on AI for diagnoses in healthcare?

                                                                B)（判断推理）

Conversation Two (Word count: 118)

M: How's your toothache?

W: It's gone, thanks. I went to the dentist last night and he took care of it.

M: Which tooth was it?

W: The last one on the upper right-hand side. It has a huge filling in it now.

M: I hate having my teeth filled. It's not just the pain I hate. It's the sound of drilling.

W: So do I. I'd rather have a tooth pulled than filled. (5. B)

M: Have you ever had one of your teeth pulled?

W: No, but the one the dentist just filled will have to come out someday. He says it can't be filled again. (6. D)

  4.　What is the dialogue mainly about?　　　　　　　　　　　　D)（主旨概括）

  5.　Which one of the following is true according to the conversation?　　B)（具体细节）

  6.　What might happen to the woman's newly-filled tooth?　　　　D)（判断推理）

Conversation Three (Word count: 107)

M: Have you seen my glasses? I can't find them anywhere.

W: Go in the bathroom and look in the mirror. (8. A)

M: You mean I've got them on. (8. A) How about that?

W: You are the most absent-minded person I have ever known.

M: I can't deny it. I'd lose my head if it wasn't attached to my shoulders.

W: I'll never forget the time you went fishing and forgot to take your rod and reel. (9. A)

M: I won't forget it either but that's not the most memorable example of my forgetfulness. (7. C)

  7.　What is the topic of the conversation?　　　　　　　　　　C)（主旨概括）

  8.　Where were the man's glasses?　　　　　　　　　　　　　A)（具体细节）

9. What did the man forget once when he went fishing?   A)（具体细节）

Conversation Four (Word count: 108)

Mr. Mahoney: My arthritis has been playing me up a bit as usual—I'm having difficulty sleeping and I'm in some pain first thing in the morning. But it's the headaches that are really getting me down, they're so painful. (11. D) Sometimes I've been sick with them literally. (12. C) I'm starting to have time off work now because of them. My wife's really worried.

Dr. Swift: I can see it's the headaches that are really bothering you, (11. D) so we can start by looking at those. We'll come back to the arthritis later, if that's OK with you. Is there anything else you want to discuss today?

Mr. Mahoney: None that I can think of.

10. What are the two speakers talking about?   C)（主旨概括）

11. What bothers the patient most?   D)（具体细节）

12. What can we learn about the patient from the conversation?   C)（具体细节）

Conversation Five (Word count: 96)

W: Ok. Last night you were supposed to read an article about human bones. Are there any comments about it?

M: Well, to begin with, I was surprised to find out that there was so much going on in bones. I always assumed they were pretty lifeless. (14. A)

W: Well, that's an assumption many people make. But the fact is bones are made of dynamic living tissue that require continuous maintenance and repair. (13. C)

M: Right. That's one of the things I found so fascinating about the article, (15. B) the way the bones repair themselves. (13. C)

13. What is the discussion mainly about?   C)（主旨概括）

14. What was the student's previous assumption about bones?   A)（具体细节）

15. What might be the best word to describe the man's attitude towards the article?   B)（判断推理）

Section B

Passage One (Word count: 149)

The food we eat seems to have produced profound effects on our health. Although science has made enormous steps in making food more fit to eat, it has, at the same time, made many foods unfit to eat. (17. C) Some research has shown that eighty percent of all human illnesses are related to diet and forty percent of cancer is related to the diet as well, especially cancer of the colon. Different cultures are more prone to contracting certain illnesses because of the food that is characteristic in these cultures. (18.A) That food is related to illness is not a new discovery. In 1945, government researchers realized that nitrates and nitrites, commonly used to preserve color in meats, and other food additives, cause cancer. Yet, these additives remain in our food, and it becomes more difficult to know which things on the packaging labels of processed food are helpful or harmful.

16. What is the best title of this passage?   D)（主旨概括）

17. Besides making food better, what else has science done to food?   C)（具体细节）

18. Why are different cultures more prone to certain illnesses?   A)（具体细节）

Passage Two (Word count: 158)

Here's a dreamy weight-loss plan: take a nap. That's the message from work by Sanjay Patel at Case Western Reserve University in Cleveland, Ohio. His study of more than 68,000 women (20. A) has found that those who sleep less than 5 hours a night gain more weight over time than those who sleep 7 hours a night. (21. A)

Controlling for other differences between the groups, Patel found that women who slept 5 hours or less gained 0.7 kilograms more on average over 10 years than 7-hour sleepers. The short-sleeping group was also 32 percent more likely to have gained 15 kilograms or more, and 15 percent more likely to have become obese.

Significantly, the short-sleepers consumed fewer calories than those who slept 7 hours, says Patel, who presented his results this week at the American Thoracic Society International Conference in San Diego, California. This finding overturns the common view that overeating among the sleep-deprived explains such weight differences.

19. What is the passage mainly about?　　　　　　　　　　　　　　B)（主旨概括）

20. How many subjects did Patel have in his study?　　　　　　　　A)（具体细节）

21. According to Patel's study, which of the following is NOT true?　　A)（具体细节）

Passage Three (Word count: 157)

Suicide is a very real risk for young people who suffer from clinical depression. In fact, during the past two years, suicide has increased among youth between the ages of 10 and 19, but there are treatments that can help. Research shows that the most effective treatment is a combination of antidepressants and talk therapy. (23. A) Antidepressants work by increasing amount of the chemical serotonin which facilitates communication between neutrons in the brain. "Antidepressants are an effective treatment for most adults but when it comes to teenagers, it's not enough." said Dr. Shelton, a psychiatrist with Vanderbilt University Medical Center. "The teenage years are full of turmoil, emotion and hormonal changes and there are family conflicts and conflicts with relationships that can contribute to distress in adolescence," Shelton said. (24. D) And antidepressant medication may not be able to deal with all of those problems. "Psychotherapy, specifically cognitive behavior theory, needs to be a part of the treatment," Shelton said.

22. What is the passage mainly concerned about?　　　　　　　　B)（主旨概括）

23. What would Dr. Shelton suggest to best solve the problem?　　A)（具体细节）

24. Which of the following doesn't contribute to adolescent depression according to Dr. Shelton?
　　　　　　　　　　　　　　　　　　　　　　　　　　　　D)（具体细节）

Passage Four (Word count: 178)

Most people think "when they are depressed, it means you feel sad," said Doctor Richard Freedman. In fact, the so-called cognitive symptoms of depression are probably the most painful for a lot of people, which are the feelings that you are useless, worthless, unlovable, no good, a loser. Those are the cognitive symptoms and the most extreme cognitive symptom, of course, is a suicidal feeling (25. C) where you feel so hopeless that you don't believe anything will get better and you are better off dead. Cognitive therapy challenges that kind of thinking. For example, say you are a depressed teen and someone at school said something critical, typically that might spin into feelings of being a complete loser. Freedman said cognitive therapy helps patients see all the times they've been successful both at school and with friends. It's completely the opposite of how you feel, so you challenge them with reality and then you correct their dysfunctional beliefs and that will actually change the way they feel," Freedman says. (27. D)

25. What is the most extreme cognitive symptom of depression?　　C)（具体细节）

26. What can we infer about the cognitive therapy?　　　　　　　D)（判断推理）

27. How does the cognitive therapy work?　　　　　　　　　　　D)（具体细节）

Passage Five (Word count: 160)

Vending machines sell many different types of items. (28. B) Some of them sell cold drinks like soda, or hot drinks like coffee or hot chocolate. Others sell candy, stamps, tickets, newspapers, and other types of small merchandise.

These machines have been successful for two reasons. They save time and they are convenient. (29. C) Merchandise sold in these machines eliminates the need for a salesclerk or cashier. In many places the customer can use the machines at any time of the day or night.

Although there are many different sizes and types of vending machines, they all work in basically the same way. The customer puts a coin into the machine and then pushes a button, pulls a lever, or opens a door to receive the merchandise. Some machines will also return change to the customer for paper money. But the basic idea is the same. Customers like to save time and are usually willing to pay a higher price for this convenience.

28. What do you know about vending machines?   B）（具体细节）

29. Why are vending machines so successful?   C）（具体细节）

30. Which of the following CANNOT be inferred from the passage?   D）（判断推理）

* * *

听力成绩分析表

项目名称	正确	错误	原因	备注
对话				
片段				
听力总分				

注：原因可分为①粗心；②走神；③懵了；④根本就听不懂。

Practice Test 8

PAPER ONE

Part Ⅰ Listening Comprehension (30%)

Section A

Directions: *In this section, you will hear five conversations. At the end of each conversation, you will hear three questions about the conversation. The question will be spoken only once. After you hear the question, read the four possible answers marked A, B, C, and D. Choose the best answer and mark the letter of your choice on the* **ANSWER SHEET**.

Sample Answer

A B ● D

Listen to the following example.

You will hear:

W: Can you tell me about yourself, please?

M: Sure, my name's Harry, 18 years old, currently studying biology and chemistry at school. As you are aware, I hope to pursue a career in medicine.

W: Harry, why do you want to be a doctor?

M: Well, everyone in my family is a doctor, so I think I can follow on nicely. (2. A)

W: Apart from treating patients, what do you think being a doctor is going to require?

M: Well, you also need to be academic and have to be an excellent communicator (3. B) with your team and the patients.

Question No. 1: What are the two speakers talking about?

You will read:

1. A. Switching to biology and chemistry.
    B. Choosing to be a family physician.
    C. Going to college.
    D. **Being a doctor.**

The correct answer is D. Mark the right answer on the **ANSWER SHEET** *as indicated below:*

1. A B C ●

Question No. 2: Why does Harry choose to be a doctor?

You will read:

2. A. **Because of his family influence.**
    B. Because of the fact that he's young.
    C. Because of the practical skills he has.
    D. Because of his love for biology and chemistry.

The correct answer is A. Mark the right answer on the **ANSWER SHEET** *as indicated below:*

2. ● B C D

Question No. 3: What is mentioned by Harry as one of the requirements for a doctor?
You will read:

3. A. A strong sense of responsibility.
    B. **Good communicative skills**.
    C. Excellent health.
    D. Great patience.

The correct answer is B. Mark the right answer on the **ANSWER SHEET** *as indicated below:*

3. A ● C D

Now let's begin with Conversation One.
Conversation One

1. A. She has a headache.
    C. She wants to chat with the doctor.
    B. Her left knee has been very painful.
    D. She wants to get a referral for a specialist.

2. A. On the outside of her knee.
    C. On the inside of her knee.
    B. On the back of her knee.
    D. On the front of her knee.

3. A. It is affecting her ability to walk and stand.
    C. It is not causing any pain at all.
    B. It is only a minor inconvenience.
    D. It is only occurring at night.

Conversation Two

4. A. He has got bowel cancer.
    C. He has got bone cancer.
    B. He has got heart disease.
    D. He has got heartburn.

5. A. To have a colonoscopy.
    C. To be put on chemotherapy.
    B. To seek a second opinion.
    D. To have his bowel removed.

6. A. Thankful.
    C. Resentful.
    B. Admiring.
    D. Respectful.

Conversation Three

7. A. For the purpose of diagnosis confirmation.
    C. For the doctor's investigation.
    B. For the possibility of legal trouble.
    D. For the patient's future use.

8. A. He has got cancer in his pancreas.
    C. He suffers from fatigue.
    B. He falls with a stomach problem.
    D. He has a loss of weight.

9. A. See a dietician.
    C. Start chemotherapy.
    B. Have an operation.
    D. Take medications for pain relief.

Conversation Four

10. A. He is having a physical checkup.
    B. He has just undergone an operation.
    C. He has just recovered from an illness.
    D. He will be discharged from the hospital this afternoon.

11. A. He got an infection in the lungs.
    C. He had his gallbladder inflamed.
    B. He was suffering from influenza.
    D. He had developed a bid kidney stone.

12. A. A lot better.
    C. Couldn't be better.
    B. Terribly awful.
    D. Okay, but a bit weak.

Conversation Five

13. A. He is a pharmacist.
    C. He is a physician.
    B. He is a visitor.
    D. He is a dieter.

14. A. Cough.
    B. Diarrhea.

    C. Headache.   D. Stomachache.

15. A. Pain-killers.   B. Cough syrup.

    C. Anti-diarrheas.   D. Indigestion tablets.

Section B

Directions: *In this section, you will hear five passages. At the end of each passage, you will hear three questions about the passage. The question will be spoken only once. After you hear the question, read the four possible answers marked A, B, C, and D. Choose the best answer and mark the letter of your choice on the* **ANSWER SHEET.**

Sample Answer

A   B   ●   D

Passage One

16. A. The demand for individuals with skills in AI research.

    B. The displacement of jobs in customer service and call centers.

    C. The need for human supervision in AI-powered systems.

    D. The potential automation of repetitive tasks.

17. A. Data analysis and interpretation.

    B. AI model engineering and maintenance.

    C. Oversight and supervision of AI systems.

    D. Customer service and call center management.

18. A. An oversupply of skilled workers in the job market.

    B. Increased competition for AI research positions.

    C. A decrease in employment opportunities in data science.

    D. A potential mismatch between demand and supply of skilled workers.

Passage Two

19. A. The hard work of TAs.   B. The president's speech.

    C. A ceremony for outstanding TAs.   D. The contribution made by TAs.

20. A. 7.   B. 10.

    C. 100.   D. 500.

21. A. Teaching assistants should get $100 more.

    B. Teaching assistants teach many classes.

    C. Teaching assistants are an important part of school.

    D. Teaching assistants should work longer.

Passage Three

22. A. Eating habits and exercise.   B. Diet.

    C. Aerobic exercise.   D. Weight control.

23. A. Beef.   B. Nuts.

    C. Avocados.   D. Potatoes.

24. A. Vegetable oil.   B. Sugar.

    C. Nuts.   D. Dairy products.

Passage Four

25. A. Students who are suffering from information anxiety.

    B. Defining information anxiety before giving tips.

    C. The information age we're living in.

    D. The balance between home life and work life.

26. A. Answer the mail.   B. Read the magazines.

    C. Sort the mail.   D. File important information.

27. A. An advisor at the university.   B. A doctor in the hospital.

    C. An assistant of a doctor.   D. A talk show speaker.

Passage Five

28. A. An introduction to a poisonous plant.

    B. A chemical acting quickly on humans' central nervous.

    C. Symptoms relating to cicutoxin.

    D. The harmfulness of water hemlock.

29. A. A poisonous plant family.   B. The hemlock family.

    C. The parsley family.   D. The carrot family.

30. A. In its hollow stem.   B. In its root.

    C. In its leaves.   D. In its flowers.

模拟答题卡

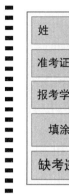

姓　名	
准考证号	
报考学校	
填涂说明	正确填涂　●　错误填涂

考生须知

1. 答题前，考生务必用黑色字迹签字笔或水笔将姓名、准考证号、报考学校填写清楚。
2. 按照题号顺序在各题目的答题区域内作答，未在对应的答题区域作答或超出答题区域的作答均不给分。
3. 选择题用2B铅笔作答，不得使用涂改液。

缺考违纪标记栏：　缺考 ◯　作弊 ◯　（此项由监考人员填涂！）

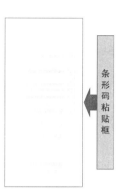

条形码粘贴框

选择题

1	(A)	(B)	(C)	(D)	16	(A)	(B)	(C)	(D)
2	(A)	(B)	(C)	(D)	17	(A)	(B)	(C)	(D)
3	(A)	(B)	(C)	(D)	18	(A)	(B)	(C)	(D)
4	(A)	(B)	(C)	(D)	19	(A)	(B)	(C)	(D)
5	(A)	(B)	(C)	(D)	20	(A)	(B)	(C)	(D)
6	(A)	(B)	(C)	(D)	21	(A)	(B)	(C)	(D)
7	(A)	(B)	(C)	(D)	22	(A)	(B)	(C)	(D)
8	(A)	(B)	(C)	(D)	23	(A)	(B)	(C)	(D)
9	(A)	(B)	(C)	(D)	24	(A)	(B)	(C)	(D)
10	(A)	(B)	(C)	(D)	25	(A)	(B)	(C)	(D)
11	(A)	(B)	(C)	(D)	26	(A)	(B)	(C)	(D)
12	(A)	(B)	(C)	(D)	27	(A)	(B)	(C)	(D)
13	(A)	(B)	(C)	(D)	28	(A)	(B)	(C)	(D)
14	(A)	(B)	(C)	(D)	29	(A)	(B)	(C)	(D)
15	(A)	(B)	(C)	(D)	30	(A)	(B)	(C)	(D)

书面表达　请用黑色签字笔在答题区域内作答，超出边框无效！

Detailed Explanations of Answers to Practice Test 8

Part I　Listening Comprehension—Tapescript and Answer Keys

Section A

Conversation One (Word count: 115)

M: Good morning, Mrs. Smith. What brings you here today?

W: Good morning, doctor. I'm here because <u>my left knee has been giving me a lot of pain lately.</u> (1. B) It's been going on for a few weeks now, and I just can't seem to shake it off.

M: I see. Can you tell me a little more about the pain? Where is it located, and does it happen all the time or only when you move a certain way?

W: <u>It's located on the inside of my knee,</u>(2. C) and <u>it hurts most when I'm walking or standing for more than a few minutes. The pain is sharp, and sometimes it feels like it's shooting down my leg. (3. A)</u>

M: OK. Please lie down on the bed, and I will have a look at your knees.

1. What is the reason for the woman's visit to the doctor?　　　　　B)（主旨概括）
2. Where is the pain located, according to the woman?　　　　　C)（具体细节）
3. What can be inferred about the woman's problem?　　　　　A)（判断推理）

Conversation Two (Word count: 179)

W: Well, <u>you'll probably have to have an operation to remove the bowel or some of it. (5. D)</u> It's too diseased to save, I'm afraid.

M: How will I go on without a bowel? How can I live without a bowel?

W: During the operation, they will fit you externally with a colostomy bag.

M: You mean a bag of shit hanging inside my clothes?

W: Well, that's perhaps an unnecessarily crude way of putting it. But broadly speaking, yes. It is sealed and odour-free. They'll show you how to empty it and change it for yourself. And nobody ever needs to know you've got one unless you tell them.

M: Well, thanks a lot. <u>Cancer of the bowel. All this time you have been prescribing me tablets for hard brain. And it turns out I've got a cancer of the bowel? (4. A)</u> <u>Oh, thanks a million. What next? How will I go on now? Will I be able to live any kind of normal life? Tell me. (6. C)</u>

4. What is wrong with the man?　　　　　A)（具体细节）
5. What does the doctor recommend the man to do?　　　　　D)（具体细节）
6. What is the man's attitude toward the doctor?　　　　　C)（判断推理）

Conversation Three (Word count: 193)

W: Mr. Scott, I like to record this consultation, <u>so you and Mrs. Scott can play back later anything that may not be clear to you today. (7. D)</u> I'm afraid that the scan results aren't very good. <u>It's likely that you've got a reoccurrence of cancer in your pancreas. (8. A)</u> That would explain why you've been feeling so tired and your loss of appetite and weight.

M: Dr. Smith, do I need surgery?

W: Surgery isn't an option of this stage. Although we cannot operate, there are still a lot we can do to help you. You've got tablets for pain relief. And we can give you something stronger if you need it. We can also start you on a course of chemotherapy to help you with your symptoms. This won't cure you but will make you feel more comfortable. It's unusual to have any unpleasant side effects with this kind of chemotherapy. <u>I'd like you to see a dietician for some advice on what you eat and to help</u>

you get your ppetite back. (9. B)

7. What is the recorded consultation for? D)（具体细节）

8. According to the doctor's diagnosis, what has happened to Mr. Scott? A)（具体细节）

9. Which of the following is NOT a suggestion for Mr. Scott? B)（具体细节）

Conversation Four (Word count: 209)

W: So, did you have a comfortable night?

M: No, not really.

W: I'm sorry to hear that, and how are you feeling at the moment?

M: A bit better. (12. D)

W: That's good. Are you having sips of water?

M: No.

W: Would you like some?

M: Well, I don't really feel like it.

W: Er...you can't drink anything at the moment.

M: The nurses have been giving me mouthwashes.

W: Yes. I think you will begin to pick up as the day goes on. And we'll carry on giving you something to ease the discomfort. Does it hurt much?

M: Well, it does when I move about.

W: Right, but the sooner we have you on the move, the quicker you start to heal. So we will have you sitting in the chair this afternoon. Enjoy the sunshine.

M: Ok. I can't say I am really looking forward to that.

W: En...You had a pretty big gallstone and the gall bladder was quite inflamed. (11. C) There was a lot of infection around it and inside it. Well, it is out now, (10. B) so no need to worry about it. It won't cause you any more trouble.

10. What's true about the man in the conversation? B)（推理判断）

11. What's wrong with the man? C)（具体细节）

12. How is the man feeling now? D)（具体细节）

Conversation Five (Word count:148)

W: What seems to be wrong?

M: I've got an upset stomach. It's pretty bad. I've been up all night with it. Now, I've got a bad headache as well.

W: I see. When did it first start?

M: When I went to bed.

W: Do you think it's something you've eaten?

M: Oh, for sure. I'm not used to all this wining and dining.

W: Yes, you've really eaten a lot.

M: You can say that again.

W: Have you got diarrhea? Is it very loose?

M: That's what it feels like.

W: How often do you have to go?

M: I have to go every few minutes.

W: Are you drinking plenty of water? Bottled water?

M: I've had a few sips of water. I feel terribly thirsty.

W: Have you taken anything? Did you bring anything from home?

M: I've got only these indigestion tablets. (15. D)

    13. Which of the following best describes the man in the dialogue?   B）（判断推理）

    14. The man suffered from the following symptoms EXCEPT_____?   A）（具体细节）

    15. What medicine did the man bring with him from home?   D）（具体细节）

Section B

Passage One (Word count: 152)

The rise of AI language models like ChatGPT has raised concerns about its potential impact on job opportunities. One of the challenges is automation. As ChatGPT becomes increasingly effective at handling customer queries and providing support, it could lead to job displacement in customer service and call center industries. (16. B) Tasks that were once performed by human agents might be taken over by intelligent AI chatbots.

Another challenge is the need for human supervision. While ChatGPT can generate human-like responses, it still requires oversight to ensure accuracy, professionalism, and adherence to ethical standards. This means that jobs may shift from being purely interactive to roles that involve monitoring and managing the AI system.

Furthermore, there is a demand for individuals with the skills to develop and maintain these AI models. Job opportunities may emerge in the field of AI research, data science, and AI model engineering. (17. B) However, there could be a mismatch between the supply of such skilled workers and the demand for these specialized roles, (18. D) which could further exacerbate job market challenges.

In short, coping with these challenges will require a thoughtful approach to strike a balance between the integration of AI into operations and safeguarding employment opportunities.

    16. What challenge does ChatGPT bring to job opportunities?   B）（主旨概括）

    17. What is one job role that may emerge with the rise of AI language models?   B）（判断推理）

    18. What could be a possible consequence of the demand for specialized AI roles?   D）（具体细节）

Passage Two (Word count: 135)

Ten graduate students who have been teaching assistants this year have been nominated to receive awards for outstanding teaching. (20. B) They were chosen from out of approximately 500 teaching assistants. There will be a ceremony on Tuesday evening at 7:30 to honor them, at which time each TA will be presented with a cash prize of $100 and a certificate commending him or her. The president recognizes that teaching assistants are an integral part of our campus, (21. C) and that the quality of undergraduate education has been improved by the quality of our TAs. They work long hours leading discussion groups, grading papers, and overseeing lab work. Most of them work as teaching assistants to help with the cost of their education. Please come to the ceremony on Tuesday to show your appreciation of these hard-working students.

    19. What's the main idea of this passage?   C）（主旨概括）

    20. How many students will get awards?   B）（具体细节）

    21. According to the speaker, what does the president think?   C）（具体细节）

Passage Three (Word count: 157)

Developing good eating habits and proper exercise is a permanent issue. (22. A) And it's the main topic of this workshop.

In order to keep a healthy diet and minimize the risk of disease, it's essential to eat a diet that consists of low-fat foods and to maximize energy with carbohydrates. Beef, nuts, oils, avocados, and most dairy products are rich in fat, so you should eat less of those; while pasta, rice, potatoes, and bread contain almost no fat and are a high energy source of complex carbohydrates. You know that too many food manufacturers use sugar to make low-fat or fat-free foods taste good, but don't worry too much about that. You don't necessarily "eat fat" by eating sugar, since sugar is an indirect fat. (24. B) When you exercise, carbohydrates are the first calories to burn. (23. D) If you want to burn off fat, it's good to do some sort of aerobic exercise such as biking, swimming, running, or fast walking.

22. What is the main topic of this talk?   A)（主旨概括）

23. According to the speaker, which one of the following will burn off the most quickly with exercise?

D)（具体细节）

24. According to the speaker, what is "indirect fat"?   B)（具体细节）

Passage Four (Word count: 146)

Through the years of being an advisor at the university, (27. A) I've often been requested to give suggestions about how to handle "information anxiety". Students come into my office who feel like they are really being hit with too much information. So let me give you some advice. First of all, what is "information anxiety"? Well, as you know, we are bombarded daily by books, magazines, newspapers, television, and radio. We are hit with bills, letters, memos, faxes, and reports. All of this can cause quite a lot of anxiety, just from the process of trying to sort it all out. (26. C) It's because we are living in the "information age" that we get this bombardment of information everyday. So today let me give you some organizing tips that should make your life easier. You can apply it to your home life, your work life, or your school life.

25. What's the speech mainly about?   B)（主旨概括）

26. According to the speaker, which of the following should the listeners do when they get their mail?

C)（具体细节）

27. Who might be the speaker?   A)（具体细节）

Passage Five (Word count: 140)

In today's class we'll talk about one of the most violently poisonous plants native to North America: water hemlock. (28. A) This plant is related to the hemlock plant that you know from history, the one that Socrates used for his lethal drink. Now one thing that is surprising is that water hemlock is a member of the parsley family, (29. C) which also includes carrots, celery, and parsnips. But this plant is so poisonous that it can even poison children who make peashooters out of its hollow stems. The active ingredient in water hemlock is cicutoxin, which can be found in all parts of the plant, but mostly in its roots. (30. B) Cicutoxin is a chemical that acts quickly on humans' central nervous systems. Within a half hour convulsions can begin, accompanied by nausea, salivation, vomiting, diarrhea, abdominal pain, dilated pupils, fever, and delirium.

28. What's the main idea of the passage?   A)（主旨概括）

29. According to the speaker, to which category does water hemlock belong?   C)（具体细节）

30. In which part of the plant is cicutoxin the most concentrated?   B)（判断推理）

* * *

听力成绩分析表

项目名称	正确	错误	原因	备注
对话				
片段				
听力总分				

注：原因可分为①粗心；②走神；③懵了；④根本就听不懂。

Practice Test 9

PAPER ONE

Part I Listening Comprehension (30%)

Section A

Directions: *In this section, you will hear five conversations. At the end of each conversation, you will hear three questions about the conversation. The question will be spoken only once. After you hear the question, read the four possible answers marked A, B, C, and D. Choose the best answer and mark the letter of your choice on the* **ANSWER SHEET**.

Sample Answer

A B ● D

Listen to the following example.

You will hear:

W: Can you tell me about yourself, please?

M: Sure, my name's Harry, 18 years old, currently studying biology and chemistry at school. As you are aware, I hope to pursue a career in medicine.

W: Harry, why do you want to be a doctor?

M: Well, everyone in my family is a doctor, so I think I can follow on nicely. (2. A)

W: Apart from treating patients, what do you think being a doctor is going to require?

M: Well, you also need to be academic and have to be an excellent communicator (3. B) with your team and the patients.

Question No. 1: What are the two speakers talking about?

You will read:

1. A. Switching to biology and chemistry.

    B. Choosing to be a family physician.

    C. Going to college.

    D. **Being a doctor.**

The correct answer is D. Mark the right answer on the **ANSWER SHEET** *as indicated below:*

1. A B C ●

Question No. 2: Why does Harry choose to be a doctor?

You will read:

2. A. **Because of his family influence.**

    B. Because of the fact that he's young.

    C. Because of the practical skills he has.

    D. Because of his love for biology and chemistry.

The correct answer is A. Mark the right answer on the **ANSWER SHEET** *as indicated below:*

2. ● B C D

Question No. 3: What is mentioned by Harry as one of the requirements for a doctor?
You will read:

3.　A. A strong sense of responsibility.

　　B. **Good communicative skills**.

　　C. Excellent health.

　　D. Great patience.

The correct answer is B. Mark the right answer on the **ANSWER SHEET** *as indicated below:*

3. A ● C D

Now let's begin with Conversation One.

Conversation One

1.　A. She is a dentist.　　　　　　　　　　B. She is an orthopaedist.

　　C. She is a physiotherapist.　　　　　　D. She is a pharmacist.

2.　A. She is examining the man.　　　　　　B. She is taking a history.

　　C. She is explaining the man's condition.　D. She is discussing a case with her colleague.

3.　A. Sliding over the stairs.　　　　　　　B. Straightening his spine.

　　C. Bending his knee too hard.　　　　　D. Lifting heavy loads in the wrong way.

Conversation Two

4.　A. The man's skin problems.　　　　　　B. The urgency of the man's problem.

　　C. The availability of the doctors.　　　D. Making an appointment with the doctor.

5.　A. With Dr. Smith at 10 on Wednesday.　B. With Dr. Smith at 10 on Tuesday.

　　C. With Dr. John at 10 on Wednesday.　D. With Dr. John at 10 on Tuesday.

6.　A. He is out of town.　　　　　　　　　B. He has a conference that day.

　　C. He is too itchy to come.　　　　　　D. Not mentioned.

Conversation Three

7.　A. On his thighs and forelegs.　　　　　B. On his thighs and forearms.

　　C. On his forearms and forelegs.　　　　D. On his forearms and forehead.

8.　A. Anemia.　　　　　　　　　　　　　　B. Influenza.

　　C. Leukemia.　　　　　　　　　　　　　D. Insomnia.

9.　A. To check the reoccurrence of the disease.　B. To determine the type of flu virus.

　　C. To prepare for blood transfusion.　　　D. To confirm the diagnosis.

Conversation Four

10.　A. Nausea.　　　　　　　　　　　　　　B. Fever.

　　C. A cold.　　　　　　　　　　　　　　D. Diarrhea.

11.　A. The stale food he ate.　　　　　　　B. The fruit juice he drank.

　　C. Too much food he ate.　　　　　　　D. The cold he got.

12.　A. Porridge.　　　　　　　　　　　　　B. Purified water.

　　C. Pizza.　　　　　　　　　　　　　　　D. Apple juice.

Conversation Five

13.　A. The wrong date of the woman's last period.　B. The weight of the baby.

　　C. The height of the baby.　　　　　　　D. The length of the woman's pregnancy.

14.　A. He is a babysitter.　　　　　　　　　B. He is an oncologist.

　　C. He is a pediatrician.　　　　　　　　D. He is an obstetrician.

15. A. 29 centimeters.   B. 32 centimeters.
    C. 19 centimeters.   D. Not mentioned.

Section B

Directions: *In this section, you will hear five passages. At the end of each passage, you will hear three questions about the passage. The question will be spoken only once. After you hear the question, read the four possible answers marked A, B, C, and D. Choose the best answer and mark the letter of your choice on the* **ANSWER SHEET.**

Sample Answer
A B ● D

Passage One

16. A. Obese people need more food.   B. Obese people require more fuel.
    C. Obesity contributes to global warming.   D. Obesity is growing as a global phenomenon.

17. A. Limited living space.
    B. Crowded shopping malls.
    C. Food shortages and higher energy prices.
    D. Incidence of diabetes and cardiovascular diseases.

18. A. Over 700 million.   B. Over 400 million.
    C. Over 2.3 billion.   D. Over 3 billion.

Passage Two

19. A. To make suggestions about proper nutrition.
    B. To report the latest breakthroughs in medical science.
    C. To talk about sleeping problems.
    D. To offer advice on how to increase one's energy.

20. A. Your heart rate increases.   B. You become even more tired.
    C. You solve the fatigue problem.   D. You'll get hungry.

21. A. Take a nap.   B. Do some work.
    C. Take a brisk walk.   D. Have a cup of coffee.

Passage Three

22. A. Eating too much.   B. Undereating.
    C. Trouble sleeping.   D. Intensive counselling.

23. A. Most of them are a result of overeating.
    B. They must be treated by hospitalization.
    C. Undereating is the most fatal among eating disorders.
    D. There is no cure for them yet.

24. A. Societal pressure.   B. Poor nutritional education.
    C. Poverty.   D. Poor health.

Passage Four

25. A. How to cope with alcoholism.   B. How to contact AA members.
    C. What causes alcoholism.   D. Why people drink.

26. A. He will not be able to see things.
    B. He cannot remember events during and after drinking.
    C. He will experience great tension.
    D. He cannot recognize friends.

27. A. Health counsellors.
    C. People who used to be problem drinkers.
    B. Volunteers who wish to help an alcoholic.
    D. Medical professionals.

Passage Five

28. A. The basic needs of men.
    C. The origin of human shelter.
    B. The first permanent shelter.
    D. The life of primitive men.

29. A. Rocks.
    C. Animal skins.
    B. Dried mud.
    D. Tree branches.

30. A. They were built by fishermen.
    C. They were built after men learned to farm.
    B. They could be easily transported.
    D. Lasting food supply is an essential factor.

Stop   **Stop**   **Stop**

模拟答题卡

姓　名	
准考证号	
报考学校	
填涂说明	正确填涂 ● 　错误填涂 ⊘ ⊗ ⊖

考生须知

1. 答题前，考生务必用黑色字迹签字笔或水笔将姓名、准考证号、报考学校填写清楚。
2. 按照题号顺序在各题目的答题区域内作答，未在对应的答题区域作答或超出答题区域的作答均不给分。
3. 选择题用2B铅笔作答，不得使用涂改液。

缺考违纪标记栏：　缺考 ○　　作弊 ○　　（此项由监考人员填涂！）

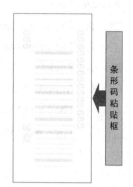

条形码粘贴框

选择题

1	(A)	(B)	(C)	(D)	16	(A)	(B)	(C)	(D)
2	(A)	(B)	(C)	(D)	17	(A)	(B)	(C)	(D)
3	(A)	(B)	(C)	(D)	18	(A)	(B)	(C)	(D)
4	(A)	(B)	(C)	(D)	19	(A)	(B)	(C)	(D)
5	(A)	(B)	(C)	(D)	20	(A)	(B)	(C)	(D)
6	(A)	(B)	(C)	(D)	21	(A)	(B)	(C)	(D)
7	(A)	(B)	(C)	(D)	22	(A)	(B)	(C)	(D)
8	(A)	(B)	(C)	(D)	23	(A)	(B)	(C)	(D)
9	(A)	(B)	(C)	(D)	24	(A)	(B)	(C)	(D)
10	(A)	(B)	(C)	(D)	25	(A)	(B)	(C)	(D)
11	(A)	(B)	(C)	(D)	26	(A)	(B)	(C)	(D)
12	(A)	(B)	(C)	(D)	27	(A)	(B)	(C)	(D)
13	(A)	(B)	(C)	(D)	28	(A)	(B)	(C)	(D)
14	(A)	(B)	(C)	(D)	29	(A)	(B)	(C)	(D)
15	(A)	(B)	(C)	(D)	30	(A)	(B)	(C)	(D)

书面表达　请用黑色签字笔在答题区域内作答，超出边框无效！

Detailed Explanations of Answers to Practice Test 9

Part I Listening Comprehension—Tapescript and Answer Keys

Section A

Conversation One (Word count: 124)

W: Well, Mr. Timpson, there is a nerve running behind your knee and your head and through your spine.

M: Aha?

W: When you lift your leg, that nerve should slide in and out of your spine quite freely. But with your leg, the nerve won't slide very far. When you lift it, the nerve gets trapped and it is very sore. When I bend your knee, that takes the tension off and eases the pain. If we straighten it, the nerve goes tight, and it's painful.

M: Ahi.

W: Now what's trapping the nerve? Well, your MRI scan confirms that you've got a damaged disc in the lower part of your back.

M: Oh. I see.

W: The disc is a little pad of gristle, which lies between the bone and your spine. (1. B) Now if you lift heavy loads in the wrong way, (3. D) you can damage it. And that's what happened to you.

  1. What does the woman most probably do?   B)（判断推理）

  2. What is the woman doing now?   C)（主旨概括）

  3. What caused damages to the man's disc?   D)（具体细节）

Conversation Two (Word count: 116)

W: Good morning, Samson's Clinic. What can I do for you?

M: I need to come in and see the doctor. I have really itchy skin and think I may have to have it looked at.

W: I have times available for Tuesday or Wednesday. Which one would work best for you? (4. D)

M: I want to come in on Wednesday. (5. A) I have a conference to attend to on Tuesday. (6. B)

W: I can fit you in on that day at 10:00. (5. A) Dr. Smith or Dr. John is available. Which of them would you prefer?

M: I would prefer Dr. Smith. (5. A)

W: OK. I will jot it down. I am looking forward to seeing you then.

M: Thanks.

  4. What is the conversation mainly about?   D)（主旨概括）

  5. What is the man's appointment?   A)（具体细节）

  6. Why can't the man come to the clinic on Tuesday?   B)（判断推理）

Conversation Three (Word count: 180)

W: What were the main problems?

M: I just got weaker and weaker. I ran out of the energy and fainted in the clinic yesterday.

W: Have you got any bruising?

M: Yes. I noticed some on my thighs and one of my forearms while I had my blood taken. (7. B)

W: Oh, dear. Any bleeding from the gums?

M: No.

W: Have you had any problem with infection recently?

M: No. Well, I had flu about two months ago.

W: Has anyone in your family had blood problems?

M: Well, my granny had anemia and was treated with ion.

W: Emmm, I was thinking of more serious blood diseases.

M: Not that I know of.

W: Are there any other things you think I should know about?

M: No. Do you think it's leukemia, doctor?

W: Well, I've still got to take more blood to confirm the diagnosis, (9. D) but I've seen the results of the previous test and I am afraid there is a 95% chance that it is leukemia. (8. C) Have you any questions before we take the extra blood?

    7. Where are the man's bruises?   B)（具体细节）

    8. What is the man most probably suffering from?   C)（判断推理）

    9. Why does the woman want to administer another blood test?   D)（判断推理）

Conversation Four (Word count: 121)

M: I feel an abdominal pain and nausea.

W: Do you feel like vomiting?

M: Yes. I also have a slight fever.

W: How about your bowel movements?

M: Since this morning, I have been passing loose and watery stools several times.

W: You are suffering from diarrhea. (10. D) What did you eat yesterday?

M: I ate some stale bread and other food. (11. A)

W: The food might have been contaminated with bacteria.

M: Can I eat or drink anything?

W: You should drink a lot of water and fruit juice. But do not eat for a day so that your bowels will have a rest. If you eat, take small servings of soft bland foods such as porridge and cereal. Avoid large meals. (12. C)

    10. What is the woman's diagnosis of the man?   D)（主旨概括）

    11. What might be the cause of the man's illness?   A)（判断推理）

    12. In order to recover soon, which of the following should the man avoid eating or drinking?

                                                          C)（具体细节）

Conversation Five (Word count: 150)

M: Now if you'd like to lie down on the couch, I'll take a look at the baby. I'll just measure to see what height it is. (13. C) Right. The baby seems slightly small.

W: How do you know that?

M: I measure from the top of your womb to your pubic bone. (14. D) The number of centimetres is roughly equal to the number of weeks you're pregnant. In your case, it's 29 centimetres but you're 32 weeks pregnant. (15. A)

W: Why do you think the baby's small?

M: It might be because your dates are wrong. Remember you weren't sure of your last period. The best thing would be to have another scan done. I'll make an appointment for you next week.

    13. What are the speakers talking about?   C)（主旨概括）

    14. What does the man do?   D)（判断推理）

    15. How long is the baby according to the doctor?   A)（具体细节）

Section B

Passage One (Word count: 156)

Global warming is also made worse by growing obesity worldwide. Obese and overweight people require more fuel to transport them and the food they eat. The problem will worsen as the population literally swells in size, a team at the London School of Hygiene & Tropical Medicine says. This adds to the food shortages and higher energy prices, (17. C) the school's researchers wrote in the journal Lancet on Friday. At least 400 million adults worldwide are obese. The World Health Organization projects by 2015, 2.3 billion adults will be overweight and more than 700 million will be obese. (18. A) In their model, the researchers pegged 40 percent of the global population as obese with a body mass index (BMI) of near 30. Many nations are fast approaching or have surpassed this level. BMI is a calculation of height to weight, and the normal range is usually considered to be 18 to 25, with more than 25 considered overweight and above 30 obese.

16. Which of the following can best describe the main idea of the talk?　　C)（主旨概括）

17. Which of the following can be made worse by the growing obese population?　　C)（具体细节）

18. According to the World Health Organization (WHO), by 2015, what would be the estimated global obese population?　　A)（具体细节）

Passage Two (Word count: 148)

Do you find yourself feeling tired all the time although you get enough sleep? Then maybe this is for you. When you're feeling weak and tired, the worst thing to do is to take a nap. It won't restore your stamina. On the contrary, what happens then is your body loses even more energy than it had before, making you even more lethargic. (20. B)

What should you do, then, at these moments when you feel so tired even though you've got enough sleep? (19. D) A cup of coffee won't help much either, as it is easy to get addicted to the caffeine. The best and most natural thing to do is to take a brisk walk. (21. C) Doctors recommend the activity because it will increase the heart rate. This increased heart rate will lead to several hours of alertness. Moreover, a regular exercise routine can make your fatigue problems disappear forever.

19. What is the main topic of this talk?　　D)（主旨概括）

20. What happens if you take a nap when you're feeling tired?　　B)（具体细节）

21. Which of the following will be suggested by the author when one feels tired despite enough sleep?

C)（判断推理）

Passage Three (Word count: 162)

You might think that the most dangerous type of eating disorder that women face involves overeating, but according to medical records, that is not the case. The majority of women who die as a result of eating problems suffer from starving themselves, commonly referred to as anorexia. (23. C)

Anorexic victims are harmed due to the scarce amounts of intake. (22. B) Their bodies can barely function. This becomes especially dangerous when their failure to remain alert occurs while driving or operating machinery. Obviously, an eating disorder of this kind is as disturbing as overeating and could put the individual in great danger.

Most anorexics suffer from a poor body image, whose primary cause is society's demand on women to be overly thin. (24. A) Although anorexia ranges in age, the majority are teenagers to women in their mid-twenties. Can we do anything about those suffering from anorexia? Hospitalization has been proven effective, and specialists suggest intensive counselling for these women to bring down their injuries and fatalities.

22. What is "anorexia" according to the speaker?   B)（判断推理）

23. According to the talk, which of the following can be said about eating disorders?   C)（判断推理）

24. According to the talk, what is the main cause of anorexia?   A)（具体细节）

Passage Four (Word count: 167)

Alcoholics do not become aware of the condition until the need for alcohol becomes so great that it affects every aspect of their lives. By that time, the person may suffer from a condition known as "a blackout". This means he or she cannot remember what events took place during or after drinking. (26. B) There is no cure for alcoholism. However, there are ways in which the alcoholic can help himself stop drinking. (25. A) First, he must face the fact that he is an alcoholic. Then he can take positive steps to work out the solution. Some hospitals open special clinics for the alcoholics to stay for a rest, nourishment and withdrawal from the use of alcohol. Another form of help for alcoholics is provided by a group called "Alcoholics Anonymous" or AA. The first step is to get the person through 90 days without alcohol. Then he is given constant moral support until he is able to stay away from drinking each and every day of his life. (27. C)

25. What is probably the topic of the talk?   A)（主旨概括）

26. What happens to someone who suffers from the so-called "blackout"?   B)（具体细节）

27. What kind of people does AA consist of ?   C)（判断推理）

Passage Five (Word count: 154)

Man has three basic needs: food, clothing and shelter. Mankind needs shelter to protect him from the weather, wild animals, insects and his enemies.

Long before man learned how to build houses, he looked for natural shelters, as the animals did. The first shelters or homes actually built by man were very simple. For his building materials, he used what he could find easily around him: rocks, tree branches, grasses, animal skins. (29. B) It was a long time, however, before man began to build permanent shelters because, until man learned to farm, he lived by hunting. And, in order to follow game, he had to be able to move from one hunting ground to another. Thus, the first man-made shelters were those that could be easily transported.

The first permanent shelters were probably built twenty to forty thousand years ago by fish-eating people who lived in one place as long as the fish supply lasted. (30. D)

28. What is the topic of the talk?   C)（主旨概括）

29. Which of the following is NOT mentioned as a building material for man's first shelters?   B)（具体细节）

30. What can be implied from the first permanent shelters?   D)（判断推理）

* * *

听力成绩分析表

项目名称	正确	错误	原因	备注
对话				
片段				
听力总分				

注：原因可分为①粗心；②走神；③懵了；④根本就听不懂。

Practice Test 10

PAPER ONE

Part I Listening Comprehension (30%)

Section A

Directions: *In this section, you will hear five conversations. At the end of each conversation, you will hear three questions about the conversation. The question will be spoken only once. After you hear the question, read the four possible answers marked A, B, C, and D. Choose the best answer and mark the letter of your choice on the* **ANSWER SHEET**.

Sample Answer

A B ● D

Listen to the following example.

You will hear:

W: Can you tell me about yourself, please?

M: Sure, my name's Harry, 18 years old, currently studying biology and chemistry at school. As you are aware, I hope to pursue a career in medicine.

W: Harry, why do you want to be a doctor?

M: Well, everyone in my family is a doctor, so I think I can follow on nicely. (2. A)

W: Apart from treating patients, what do you think being a doctor is going to require?

M: Well, you also need to be academic and have to be an excellent communicator (3. B) with your team and the patients.

Question No. 1: What are the two speakers talking about?

You will read:

1. A. Switching to biology and chemistry.
   B. Choosing to be a family physician.
   C. Going to college.
   D. **Being a doctor.**

The correct answer is D. Mark the right answer on the **ANSWER SHEET** *as indicated below:*

1. A B C ●

Question No. 2: Why does Harry choose to be a doctor?

You will read:

2. A. **Because of his family influence.**
   B. Because of the fact that he's young.
   C. Because of the practical skills he has.
   D. Because of his love for biology and chemistry.

The correct answer is A. Mark the right answer on the **ANSWER SHEET** *as indicated below:*

2. ● B C D

Question No. 3: What is mentioned by Harry as one of the requirements for a doctor?

You will read:

3. A. A strong sense of responsibility.

    B. **Good communicative skills**.

    C. Excellent health.

    D. Great patience.

The correct answer is B. Mark the right answer on the **ANSWER SHEET** *as indicated below:*

3. A ● C D

Now let's begin with Conversation One.

Conversation One

1. A. The emergence of ChatGPT in the medical field.

    B. The accuracy of AI in medical diagnosis.

    C. Patients' over-dependence on AI for self-treatment.

    D. The risk of delays in seeking medical care.

2. A. Over-dependence on professionals.   B. Misdiagnosis and delayed treatment.

    C. Unreliable treatment.   D. Inaccurate self-treatment.

3. A. Limiting patient access to AI resources.

    B. Completely relying on AI for medical advice.

    C. Discarding the use of AI in self-diagnosis.

    D. Consulting professionals alongside AI tools.

Conversation Two

4. A. His low-sodium diet.   B. His high blood pressure.

    C. The university nutritionist.   D. A note given by the women.

5. A. A nutritionist.   B. A professor.

    C. A dining hall manager.   D. A doctor.

6. A. The man is a university nutritionist.

    B. The woman gives the man a note.

    C. The man can have at most three grams of sodium a day.

    D. The man can have at least three grams of sodium a day.

Conversation Three

7. A. The cause of laughter.   B. The purpose of laughter.

    C. Who and when people laugh.   D. The origins of laughter.

8. A. She feels boring to watch the movie.   B. People have found out why primates laugh.

    C. He likes to know why people like to laugh.   D. She has done a scientific research.

9. A. Doctor and patient.   B. Friends.

    C. Parent and child.   D. Employer and employee.

Conversation Four

10. A. Her injured ankle.   B. Her bad sleep.

    C. Her naughty children.   D. Her big house.

11. A. Six days ago.   B. Four hours ago.

    C. Yesterday.   D. Last week.

12. A. She has difficulty resting.   B. She has five children.

    C. She hasn't followed the doctor's advice.   D. Her leg is swollen.

Conversation Five

13. A. Causes of illness.
    C. The history of prescription drugs.
    B. The discovery of antibiotics.
    D. The strength of antibiotics.

14. A. Her lab notes.
    C. A homework assignment.
    B. A medical reference book.
    D. The name of her doctor.

15. A. To give an example of a bad reaction to penicillin.
    B. To show how penicillin has changed over the years.
    C. To emphasize the importance of antibiotics.
    D. To explain why penicillin requires a prescription.

Section B

Directions: *In this section, you will hear five passages. At the end of each passage, you will hear three questions about the passage. The question will be spoken only once. After you hear the question, read the four possible answers marked A, B, C, and D. Choose the best answer and mark the letter of your choice on the* **ANSWER SHEET.**

Sample Answer

A B ● D

Passage One

16. A. Headaches.
    C. Respiratory problems.
    B. Insomnia.
    D. Digestive problems.

17. A. On Monday in Edinburgh.
    C. On Monday at Staffordshire.
    B. On Wednesday at Edinburgh.
    D. On Wednesday at Staffordshire.

18. A. 94.
    C. 130.
    B. 41.
    D. 135.

Passage Two

19. A. Too much texting can make you shallow.
    B. Texting is nothing but a wonder of technology.
    C. Texting has more disadvantages than advantages.
    D. Too much texting results in poorly performing students.

20. A. Simply from the contents of their texts.
    C. Merely from the books they read at leisure.
    B. Just from the number of texts they send.
    D. Right from the way they spell certain words.

21. A. 2,030 sociology students.
    C. 2,030 psychology students.
    B. 2,300 sociology students.
    D. 2,300 psychology students.

Passage Three

22. A. Exercise: Value beyond Weight Loss.
    C. Exercise for a Better Life.
    B. Exercise: the Way to Well-being.
    D. Exercise for Weight Loss.

23. A. A 12-week weight loss program.
    C. A 12-week aerobic exercise program.
    B. A 12-month weight loss program.
    D. A 12-month aerobic exercise program.

24. A. Exercise sometimes is just futile and not beneficial.
    B. Exercise should be encouraged, weight loss less emphasized.
    C. Aerobic exercise can do good to people both mentally and physically.
    D. Poor weight loss can inevitably result in disappointment and low self-esteem.

Passage Four

25. A. Song sparrows take good care of their babies.

    B. Young song sparrows lack the skills and experience of their parents.

    C. There are different kinds of song sparrows in different seasons.

    D. Young and old song sparrows experience climate change differently.

26. A. Science.   B. Global Change Biology.

    C. Conservation Science.   D. Climate Change and Animals.

27. A. In the warmer spring.   B. In the hottest summer.

    C. In the coldest winter.   D. In the coolest autumn.

Passage Five

28. A. The prevention of illness.   B. A new kind of insect repellent.

    C. Poisonous chemicals in the new product.   D. The importance of taking vitamins.

29. A. It does not require a doctor.   B. It can be used by young and old people alike.

    C. It can be taken as often as needed.   D. It uses natural ingredients.

30. A. Vitamins.   B. Body temperature.

    C. More meat on the skin.   D. Certain human odors.

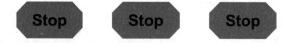

模拟答题卡

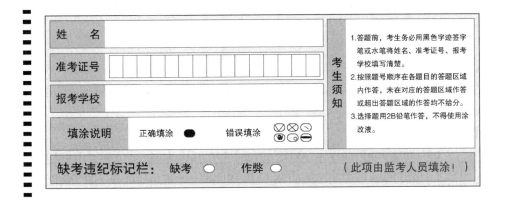

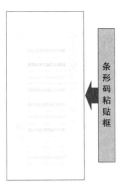

选择题	1	(A)	(B)	(C)	(D)	16	(A)	(B)	(C)	(D)
	2	(A)	(B)	(C)	(D)	17	(A)	(B)	(C)	(D)
	3	(A)	(B)	(C)	(D)	18	(A)	(B)	(C)	(D)
	4	(A)	(B)	(C)	(D)	19	(A)	(B)	(C)	(D)
	5	(A)	(B)	(C)	(D)	20	(A)	(B)	(C)	(D)
	6	(A)	(B)	(C)	(D)	21	(A)	(B)	(C)	(D)
	7	(A)	(B)	(C)	(D)	22	(A)	(B)	(C)	(D)
	8	(A)	(B)	(C)	(D)	23	(A)	(B)	(C)	(D)
	9	(A)	(B)	(C)	(D)	24	(A)	(B)	(C)	(D)
	10	(A)	(B)	(C)	(D)	25	(A)	(B)	(C)	(D)
	11	(A)	(B)	(C)	(D)	26	(A)	(B)	(C)	(D)
	12	(A)	(B)	(C)	(D)	27	(A)	(B)	(C)	(D)
	13	(A)	(B)	(C)	(D)	28	(A)	(B)	(C)	(D)
	14	(A)	(B)	(C)	(D)	29	(A)	(B)	(C)	(D)
	15	(A)	(B)	(C)	(D)	30	(A)	(B)	(C)	(D)

书面表达　请用黑色签字笔在答题区域内作答,超出边框无效!

Detailed Explanations of Answers to Practice Test 10

Part I   Listening Comprehension—Tapescript and Answer Keys
Section A
Conversation One (Word count: 120)

M: Hey Jennie, I wanted to discuss a concern about ChatGPT in the medical field from yesterday's conference, but we ran out of time.

W: What's the issue, Davis?

M: Some doctors worry patients may rely heavily on AI for self-diagnosis and treatment recommendations. (1. C) This could be risky, leading to misdiagnosis or delays in seeking proper medical care. (2. B)

W: Emphasizing consulting qualified professionals alongside AI tools is crucial. (3. D) We shouldn't replace them entirely.

M: Absolutely. We need to strike the right balance and educate patients about the limitations of AI while encouraging professional advice for accuracy.

W: Education and awareness are key to safe and effective AI use in healthcare.

M: Agreed, let's promote a collaborative approach with AI and medical expertise.

   1. What is the concern discussed by the two speakers?   C)（主旨概括）

   2. What is one potential risk of relying solely on AI for medical advice?   B)（具体细节）

   3. What do the two speakers recommend regarding the use of AI in medical care?   D)（判断推理）

Conversation Two (Word count: 106)

M: I'm looking for Mrs. O'Reilly's office.

W: I'm Mrs. O'Reilly. Come right in.

M: I was at the Student Health Services yesterday. They told me that my blood pressure is too high. (4. B)

W: Then I suppose you need a low-sodium diet to help bring your blood pressure down.

M: That's right. The doctor told me to see the university nutritionist about it, so here I am. (5. D) He gave me this note for you.

W: Let's see. It says here that you can have up to three grams of sodium a day. (6. C)

   4. What are the speakers talking about?   B)（主旨概括）

   5. Who told the man to talk to Mrs. O'Reilly?   D)（具体细节）

   6. Which of the following is true according to the conversation?   C)（具体细节）

Conversation Three (Word count: 88)

M: Well, you seemed to be having fun watching the movie?

W: Yeah, it was good fun. I think it kept me in stitches right from the start.

M: You know, whenever I watch comedy, I always like to know why it is that people like to laugh. I mean, why does it feel so good to laugh? (7. A) (8. C)

W: Yeah, I heard from my biology professor that even after centuries of scientific research, no one knows for sure why human beings and just a few other primates laugh.

   7. What is the main issue being discussed throughout?   A)（主旨概括）

   8. Which of the following is true according to the conversation?   C)（具体细节）

   9. What is the possible relationship between the two speakers?   B)（推理判断）

Conversation Four (Word count: 94)

M: Oh, it's you, Mrs. Bramley. Come in and sit down. Now, what was it? Oh, yes, your ankle. <u>Has there been any improvement since last week</u>? (11. D)

W: Well, no. I'm afraid not, doctor. The leg's still the same.

M: I'd better have another look at it. Hm. It's still very swollen. Have you been resting it, as I told you to?

W: It's so difficult to rest it, doctor, you know, with a house to run, <u>and six children and</u>...(12. B)

   10. What is the conversation mainly about? A)（主旨概括）

   11. When did the woman see the man last time? D)（具体细节）

   12. Which of the following is wrong with the woman? B)（具体细节）

Conversation Five (Word count: 113)

W: <u>Hi, Dan, you know that lab you missed? You can have my notes.</u> (14. A)

M: Thanks. I appreciate that.

W: So, how are you feeling?

M: Much better now that I am taking an antibiotic. Student Health gave me one, and it's really a help. You know what amazes me is that the human race survived before antibiotics.

W: I agree. When my father was a young boy in the 1940's, he got blood poisoning and would have died. But his doctor had heard of this new drug, called "penicillin".

M: Wow, he was really lucky. And now we have lots of antibiotics that kill bacteria.

   13. What are the speakers talking about? D)（主旨概括）

   14. What does the woman offer to give the man? A)（具体细节）

   15. Why does the woman tell the story about her father? C)（推理判断）

Section B

Passage One (Word count: 169)

Keeping a diary is bad for your health, say UK psychologists. They found that <u>people who regularly keep a diary suffer from headaches, sleeplessness, digestive problems and social awkwardness</u> (16. C) more than people who don't. This finding challenges the assumption that people find it easier to get over a traumatic event if they write about it.

"We expected that diary keepers to have more benefits or be the same but they were worst off," says Elaine Duncan of Glasgow Caledonia University."In fact, you will be probably be much better off if you don't write anything at all," she adds.

The study carried out with David Shefield of Staffordshire University was presented <u>on Wednesday at a meeting of the British Psychological Society at Edinburgh.</u> (17. B) <u>The peer studied 94 regular diarists, and compared their health with that of 41 non-diarists.</u> (18. D) The subjects, all students at Staffordshire University, answered questions about their diary keeping habits and filled in a standard questionnaire....

   16. According to UK psychologists, regular diarists are more likely to suffer from the following EXCEPT_____. C)（具体细节）

   17. When and where was the Duncan study presented? B)（具体细节）

   18. How many subjects were there in Duncan's study? D)（具体细节）

Passage Two (Word count: 139)

Teenagers who text for more than 100 times a day tend to be more shallow, image-obsessed and driven by wealth, not to mention the pretty bad spelling. The study from the University of Winnipeg suggests that a lot can be learned about a person's personality simply from the number of texts they send. The most incessant texters often turn out to be slightly more racist than others. <u>The data was gathered over a period of three years</u>

from 2,300 psychology students at the University of Winnipeg. (21. D) The theory the university study tried to test was that constant use of twitter and texting for communication results in a world where people have quick and shallow thoughts. The results indicate that students who text frequently place less importance on moral, aesthetic and spiritual goals and greater importance on wealth and image. (20. B)

19. What is the main idea of this talk?　　A)（主旨概括）
20. According to the study, how can we learn about a person's personality?　　B)（判断推理）
21. Who are the participants of the study?　　D)（具体细节）

Passage Three (Word count: 157)

Many, if not most, people start exercising because they want to lose weight. But very often they abandon exercise when they expected pounds fail to fall off. Study after study has found that, without major changes in eating habits, increasing physical activities is only somewhat effective for losing weight, though it helps people maintain weight loss, and shedding a few pounds, especially around one's middle, can improve health. For example, researchers in Brisbane, Australia, studied 58 sedentary overweight or obese men and women, who participated in a closely monitored 12-week aerobic exercise program. (23. C) Weight loss was minimal, but nonetheless participants' waistline shrunk, their blood pressure and resting heart rate dropped, and their aerobic capacity and mood improved. Exercise should be encouraged and the emphasis on weight loss reduced, the researchers concluded. (24. B) Disappointment and low self-esteem associated with poor weight loss could lead to low exercise adherence and the general perception that exercise is futile and not beneficial.

22. What can be the best topic of this talk?　　A)（主旨概括）
23. What kind of program did the participants of the study attend?　　C)（具体细节）
24. What is the conclusion reached by the researchers of the Brisbane study?　　B)（判断推理）

Passage Four (Word count: 162)

What's good for adults is not always best for the young, and vice versa. At least that is the case with song sparrows and how they experience the effects of climate change, according to two recent studies by scientists at the University of California, Davis, and Point Blue Conservation Science.

Both studies show the importance of considering the various stages and ages of individuals in a species—from babies to juveniles to adults—to best predict not only how climate change could affect a species as a whole, but also why.

In the study published in print today in the journal *Global Change Biology*, (26. B) climate change had opposite projected effects for adult and juvenile song sparrows in central coastal California. The researchers found, not surprisingly, that adult survival was sensitive to cold winter weather. (27. C)

Even though we rarely see freezing temperatures on the coast of California, it was clear that an adult bird's chances of survival were lowest in the coldest winters.

25. What is the main idea of this talk?　　D)（主旨概括）
26. In which of the following journals the study was published?　　B)（具体细节）
27. When was the lowest chances of survival for the adult sparrows?　　C)（判断推理）

Passage Five (Word count: 162)

The news is in: we have another weapon against mosquitoes. (28. B) Researchers in a pharmaceutical firm in Long Beach, California, have discovered a way to keep these irritating pests away. And it's just a pill the size of an ordinary vitamin, no toxic chemical ingredients and of course no need for shots.

The researchers argue that this method involves no risk to the body, since the pills contain only natural ingredients. (29. D) They only require purchasing the pill at a local drugstore and taking one when needed, and they last four hours. Mosquitoes are attracted to higher body temperatures, fleshier skin, and certain human smells. (30. A) The new pill causes the body to release an odor that repels mosquitoes. Unlike chemical sprays, however, that have odors perceptible to humans, the odor released by the pill cannot be detected by anyone, except the annoying pest itself. The odor released by the body is a natural odor that the body produces automatically when exposed to certain nutrients.

28. What is the main topic of the talk? B)（主旨概括）

29. Why is this method not harmful? D)（判断推理）

30. Which of the following does NOT attract mosquitoes? A)（具体细节）

* * *

听力成绩分析表

项目名称	正确	错误	原因	备注
对话				
片段				
听力总分				

注：原因可分为①粗心；②走神；③懵了；④根本就听不懂。

Part Ⅲ　Hi-Fi FATMD Tests

高仿真 FATMD 测试

国家医学考试中心标准答题卡

姓 名	
准考证号	
报考学校	

考生须知

1.答题前,考生务必用黑色字迹签字笔或水笔将姓名、准考证号、报考学校填写清楚。
2.按照题号顺序在各题目的答题区域内作答,未在对应的答题区域作答或超出答题区域的作答均不给分。
3.选择题用2B铅笔作答,不得使用涂改液。

条形码粘贴框

填涂说明　正确填涂 ●　错误填涂 ⊘⊗⊖⊘

缺考违纪标记栏：　缺考 ○　　作弊 ○　　（此项由监考人员填涂！）

选择题

1	ⒶⒷⒸⒹⒺ	16	ⒶⒷⒸⒹⒺ	31	ⒶⒷⒸⒹⒺ	46	ⒶⒷⒸⒹⒺ	61	ⒶⒷⒸⒹⒺ	76	ⒶⒷⒸⒹⒺ
2	ⒶⒷⒸⒹⒺ	17	ⒶⒷⒸⒹⒺ	32	ⒶⒷⒸⒹⒺ	47	ⒶⒷⒸⒹⒺ	62	ⒶⒷⒸⒹⒺ	77	ⒶⒷⒸⒹⒺ
3	ⒶⒷⒸⒹⒺ	18	ⒶⒷⒸⒹⒺ	33	ⒶⒷⒸⒹⒺ	48	ⒶⒷⒸⒹⒺ	63	ⒶⒷⒸⒹⒺ	78	ⒶⒷⒸⒹⒺ
4	ⒶⒷⒸⒹⒺ	19	ⒶⒷⒸⒹⒺ	34	ⒶⒷⒸⒹⒺ	49	ⒶⒷⒸⒹⒺ	64	ⒶⒷⒸⒹⒺ	79	ⒶⒷⒸⒹⒺ
5	ⒶⒷⒸⒹⒺ	20	ⒶⒷⒸⒹⒺ	35	ⒶⒷⒸⒹⒺ	50	ⒶⒷⒸⒹⒺ	65	ⒶⒷⒸⒹⒺ	80	ⒶⒷⒸⒹⒺ
6	ⒶⒷⒸⒹⒺ	21	ⒶⒷⒸⒹⒺ	36	ⒶⒷⒸⒹⒺ	51	ⒶⒷⒸⒹⒺ	66	ⒶⒷⒸⒹⒺ	81	ⒶⒷⒸⒹⒺ
7	ⒶⒷⒸⒹⒺ	22	ⒶⒷⒸⒹⒺ	37	ⒶⒷⒸⒹⒺ	52	ⒶⒷⒸⒹⒺ	67	ⒶⒷⒸⒹⒺ	82	ⒶⒷⒸⒹⒺ
8	ⒶⒷⒸⒹⒺ	23	ⒶⒷⒸⒹⒺ	38	ⒶⒷⒸⒹⒺ	53	ⒶⒷⒸⒹⒺ	68	ⒶⒷⒸⒹⒺ	83	ⒶⒷⒸⒹⒺ
9	ⒶⒷⒸⒹⒺ	24	ⒶⒷⒸⒹⒺ	39	ⒶⒷⒸⒹⒺ	54	ⒶⒷⒸⒹⒺ	69	ⒶⒷⒸⒹⒺ	84	ⒶⒷⒸⒹⒺ
10	ⒶⒷⒸⒹⒺ	25	ⒶⒷⒸⒹⒺ	40	ⒶⒷⒸⒹⒺ	55	ⒶⒷⒸⒹⒺ	70	ⒶⒷⒸⒹⒺ	85	ⒶⒷⒸⒹⒺ
11	ⒶⒷⒸⒹⒺ	26	ⒶⒷⒸⒹⒺ	41	ⒶⒷⒸⒹⒺ	56	ⒶⒷⒸⒹⒺ	71	ⒶⒷⒸⒹⒺ	86	ⒶⒷⒸⒹⒺ
12	ⒶⒷⒸⒹⒺ	27	ⒶⒷⒸⒹⒺ	42	ⒶⒷⒸⒹⒺ	57	ⒶⒷⒸⒹⒺ	72	ⒶⒷⒸⒹⒺ	87	ⒶⒷⒸⒹⒺ
13	ⒶⒷⒸⒹⒺ	28	ⒶⒷⒸⒹⒺ	43	ⒶⒷⒸⒹⒺ	58	ⒶⒷⒸⒹⒺ	73	ⒶⒷⒸⒹⒺ	88	ⒶⒷⒸⒹⒺ
14	ⒶⒷⒸⒹⒺ	29	ⒶⒷⒸⒹⒺ	44	ⒶⒷⒸⒹⒺ	59	ⒶⒷⒸⒹⒺ	74	ⒶⒷⒸⒹⒺ	89	ⒶⒷⒸⒹⒺ
15	ⒶⒷⒸⒹⒺ	30	ⒶⒷⒸⒹⒺ	45	ⒶⒷⒸⒹⒺ	60	ⒶⒷⒸⒹⒺ	75	ⒶⒷⒸⒹⒺ	90	ⒶⒷⒸⒹⒺ

书 面 表 达　　请用黑色签字笔在答题区域内作答,超出黑色边框区域的答案无效!

样张（英语）

5

10

国家医学考试中心监制　　　　　北京世纪互联软件开发有限公司设计制作　LT-1/8L 2019L146F

书 面 表 达　　　　请用黑色签字笔在答题区域内作答，超出黑色边框区域的答案无效！

15

20

25

30

LT-1/8R 2013B002B

Hi-Fi FATMD Test 1

PAPER ONE

Part I Listening Comprehension (30%)

Section A

Directions: *In this section, you will hear five conversations. At the end of each conversation, you will hear three questions about the conversation. The question will be spoken only once. After you hear the question, read the four possible answers marked A, B, C, and D. Choose the best answer and mark the letter of your choice on the* **ANSWER SHEET**.

Sample Answer

A B ● D

Listen to the following example.

You will hear:

W: Can you tell me about yourself, please?

M: Sure, my name's Harry, 18 years old, currently studying biology and chemistry at school. As you are aware, I hope to pursue a career in medicine.

W: Harry, why do you want to be a doctor?

M: Well, everyone in my family is a doctor, so I think I can follow on nicely. (2. A)

W: Apart from treating patients, what do you think being a doctor is going to require?

M: Well, you also need to be academic and have to be an excellent communicator (3. B) with your team and the patients.

Questions number 1 to 3 are based on the conversation you have just heard.

Question No. 1: What are the two speakers talking about?

You will read:

1. A. Switching to biology and chemistry.   B. Choosing to be a family physician.
    C. Going to college.   D. **Being a doctor.**

The correct answer is D. Mark the right answer on the **ANSWER SHEET** *as indicated below:*

1. A B C ●

Question No. 2: Why does Harry choose to be a doctor?

You will read:

2. A. **Because of his family influence.**

    B. Because of the fact that he's young.

    C. Because of the practical skills he has.

    D. Because of his love for biology and chemistry.

The correct answer is A. Mark the right answer on the **ANSWER SHEET** *as indicated below:*

2. ● B C D

Question No. 3: What is mentioned by Harry as one of the requirements for a doctor?

You will read:

3. A. A strong sense of responsibility. **B. Good communicative skills.**
    C. Excellent health. D. Great patience.

The correct answer is B. Mark the right answer on the **ANSWER SHEET** *as indicated below:*

3. A ● C D

Now let's begin with Conversation One.

Conversation One

1. A. He might have a stroke. B. He has a drinking problem.
    C. He might have a heart attack. D. His blood pressure is slightly high.
2. A. Take diuretics. B. Take beta-blocks.
    C. Give up alcohol soon. D. Change his life-style.
3. A. Flushing out extra fluid and salt in the body.
    B. Helping the patient to lose some weight.
    C. Blocking the effects of adrenalin on the heart.
    D. Reducing the amount of stress to the heart.

Conversation Two

4. A. Medical specialist and a patient. B. A general practitioner and a patient.
    C. A doctor and an interne. D. A doctor and a nurse.
5. A. Her heavy smoking. B. Her heavy sputum.
    C. Her worries about work. D. Her persistent cough.
6. A. How she lost her job. B. Her cough and her other symptoms.
    C. How she tried to quit smoking. D. Why she has so many health problems.

Conversation Three

7. A. Because he has pneumonia. B. Because his wife told him to.
    C. Because he feels tired. D. Because his wife feels tired.
8. A. A few days. B. Four years.
    C. Six months. D. Two weeks.
9. A. When the doctor told him to. B. When his wife told him to.
    C. When he had to. D. When he felt better.

Conversation Four

10. A. She has difficulty with her present job.
    B. She wants to get rid of her chest infection.
    C. The antibiotic doesn't work for her and has some side effects.
    D. She is worried about losing her job.
11. A. Thrush. B. Exhausted.
    C. Still feeling bad after taking the antibiotics. D. Insomnia.
12. A. The antibiotic doesn't fit the patient. B. The side effect takes time to disappear.
    C. The patient doesn't complete the course. D. The patient works for too long a time.

Conversation Five

13. A. He is infected with HIV. B. He has depression.
    C. He is an insomniac. D. He has diabetes.
14. A. His sister might be infected because he is close to her.
    B. He doesn't have a friend to talk to about his problem.

C. A friend of his died of AIDS.

D. He has been exposed to H1N1 virus.

15. A. A friend of his. B. His sister.

C. One of his colleagues. D. His father.

Section B

Directions: *In this section, you will hear five passages. At the end of each passage, you will hear three questions about the passage. The question will be spoken only once. After you hear the question, read the four possible answers labelled A, B, C, and D. Choose the best answer and mark the letter of your choice on the* **ANSWER SHEET.**

Sample Answer

A B ● D

Passage One

16. A. Patients from foreign countries. B. Medical internes and residents.

C. Students of English. D. Patients with little knowledge of English.

17. A. The importance of language in cross-cultural communication.

B. English, an obstacle in cross-cultural medical communication.

C. English, a key to cross-cultural medical communication.

D. Language in cross-cultural communication in medicine.

18. A. It might arouse inappropriate behavior in the patient.

B. It might give pressures to the doctor and the patient.

C. It might harm doctor-patient relationship and the care.

D. It might make the patient angry and depressed.

Passage Two.

19. A. How to protect against heart disease. B. How to run for your health.

C. Differences between runners and non-runners. D. How running helps one live longer.

20. A. More than 3,400. B. About one-fourth.

C. About 1,200. D. 55,000.

21. A. Runners had a much higher risk of death than non-runners.

B. Runners had a lower risk of death than non-runners by 30%.

C. Runners had a lower risk of death than non-runners by 45%.

D. Runners had a lower risk of death than non-runners by 25%.

Passage Three

22. A. Chronic illness. B. Loss of independence.

C. Ever-increasing frailty. D. Worsening memory.

23. A. Abilities of daily living. B. Activities of daily learning.

C. Abilities of daily learning. D. Activities of daily living.

24. A. How to have a doctor-patient conversation.

B. How to take care of older patients without independence.

C. How to take a medical history of older patients.

D. How to assess the daily activities of older patients.

Passage Four

25. A. How to ask patients about their medical history.

B. How to coax patients into talking about their medical history.

    C. How to pick out useful information from patients' medical history.

    D. Patients having difficulty recalling their medical history.

26. A. Doing a little coaxing.

    B. Beginning with an open question and moving on to closed ones.

    C. Interrogating or bombarding the patient with questions.

    D. Allowing the patient time to reflect before moving on to the next step.

27. A. They may forget their illnesses that happened years ago.

    B. They are reluctant to recall their previous traumatic events.

    C. They choose to forget the recent death in their family.

    D. They don't have problems recalling their recent illnesses.

Passage Five

28. A. Before an operation.   B. After a ward round.

    C. After a rotation.   D. Before the patient was admitted.

29. A. For myocardial infarction.   B. For confusion and increased nocturia.

    C. For serious chest infection.   D. For respiratory tract infection.

30. A. About 4 days after the GP's first visit.   B. About 2 days after the GP's first visit.

    C. About 2 weeks after the GP's first visit.   D. About 24 hours after the GP's first visit.

Part Ⅱ　Vocabulary (10%)

Section A

Directions: *In this section, all the sentences are incomplete. Four words or phrases marked A, B, C, and D are given beneath each of them. You are to choose the word or phrase that best completes the sentence. Then, mark your answer on the* **ANSWER SHEET**.

31. Chronic high-dose intake of vitamin A has been shown to have _____ effects on bone.

    A. adverse   B. prevalent   C. instant   D. purposeful

32. Drinking more water is good for the rest of your body, helping to lubricate joints and _____ toxins and impurities.

    A. screen out   B. knock out   C. flush out   D. rule out

33. The rheumatologist advises that those with ongoing aches and pains first seek medical help to _____ the problem.

    A. affiliate   B. alleviate   C. aggravate   D. accelerate

34. Generally, vaccine makers _____ the virus in fertilized chicken eggs in a process that can take four to six months.

    A. penetrate   B. designate   C. generate   D. exaggerate

35. Danish research shows that the increase in obese people in Denmark is roughly _____ to the increase of carbon dioxide in the atmosphere.

    A. equivalent   B. temporary   C. permanent   D. relevant

36. Ted was felled by a massive stroke that affected his balance and left him barely able to speak _____.

    A. bluntly   B. intelligibly   C. reluctantly   D. ironically

37. In a technology-intensive enterprise, computers _____ all processes of the production and management.

    A. dominate   B. overwhelm   C. substitute   D. imitate

38. Although most dreams apparently happen _____, dream activity may be provided by external influences.

A. homogeneously B. instantaneously C. spontaneously D. simultaneously

39. We are much quicker to respond, and we respond far too quickly by giving _____ to our anger.

    A. vent B. impulse C. temper D. offence

40. By maintaining a strong family _____, they are also maintaining the infrastructure of society.

    A. bias B. honor C. estate D. bond

Section B

Directions: *Each of the following sentences has a word or phrase underlined. Beneath each sentence, there are four words or phrases marked A, B, C, and D. Choose the word or phrase which can best keep the meaning of the original sentence if it is substituted for the underlined part. Mark the letter of your choice on the **ANSWER SHEET**.*

41. Inform the manager that you are on medication that makes you drowsy.

    A. uneasy B. sleepy C. guilty D. fiery

42. Diabetes is one of the most prevalent and potentially dangerous diseases in the world.

    A. crucial B. virulent C. colossal D. widespread

43. Likewise, soot and smoke from fire contain a multitude of carcinogens.

    A. a matter of B. a body of C. plenty of D. sort of

44. Many questions about estrogen's effects remain to be elucidated, and investigators are seeking answers through ongoing laboratory and clinical studies.

    A. implicated B. implies C. illuminated D. initiated

45. A network chatting is a limp substitute for meeting friends over coffee.

    A. accomplishment B. refreshment C. complement D. replacement

46. When patients spend extended periods in hospitals, they tend to become overly dependent and lose interest in taking care of themselves.

    A. extremely B. exclusively C. exactly D. explicitly

47. Attempts to restrict parking in the city centre have further aggravated the problem of the traffic congestion.

    A. ameliorated B. aggregated C. deteriorated D. duplicated

48. It was reported that bacteria contaminated up to 80% of domestic retail raw chicken in the United States.

    A. inflamed B. inflicted C. infected D. infiltrated

49. Researchers recently ran the numbers on gun violence in the United States and reported that right-to-carry-gun laws do not inhibit violent crime.

    A. curb B. induce C. lessen D. impel

50. Regardless of our uneasiness about stereotypes, numerous studies have shown clear differences between Chinese and western parenting.

    A. specification B. sensations C. conventions D. conservations

Part Ⅲ Cloze (10%)

Directions: *In this section, there is a passage with ten numbered blanks. For each blank, there are four choices marked A, B, C, and D on the right side. Choose the best answer and mark the letter of your choice on the **ANSWER SHEET**.*

It was the kind of research that gave insight into how flu strains could mutate so quickly. (One theory behind the 1918 version's sudden demise after wreaking so much devastation was that it mutated to a nonlethal form.) The same branch of research concluded in 2005 that the 1918 flu started in birds before passing to humans. Parsing this animal-human __51__ could provide clues to __52__ the next potential superflu, which already has a name: H5N1, also known as avian flu or bird flu.

This potential killer also has a number: 59%. According to the WHO, nearly three-fifths of the people who __53__ H5N1 since 2003 died from the virus, which was first reported __54__ humans in Hong Kong in 1997 before a more serious __55__ occurred in Southeast Asia between 2003 and 2004. Some researchers argue that those mortality numbers are exaggerated because WHO only __56__ cases in which victims are sick enough to go to the hospital for treatment. __57__, compare that to the worldwide mortality rate of the 1918 pandemic; it may have killed roughly 50 million people, but that was only 10 percent of the number of people infected, according to a 2006 estimate.

H5N1's saving grace—and the only reason we're not running around masked up in public right now—is that the strain doesn't jump from birds to humans, or from humans to humans, easily. There have been just over 600 cases (and 359 deaths) since 2003. But __58__ its lethality, and the chance it could turn into something far more transmissible, one might expect H5N1 research to be exploding, with labs __59__ the virus's molecular components to understand how it spreads between animals and __60__ to humans, and hoping to discover a vaccine that could head off a pandemic.

51. A. rejection B. interface
    C. complement D. contamination
52. A. be stopped B. stopping
    C. being stopped D. having stopped
53. A. mutated B. effected
    C. infected D. contracted
54. A. in B. on
    C. with D. from
55. A. trigger B. launch
    C. outbreak D. outcome
56. A. counts B. amounts to
    C. accounts to D. accumulates
57. A. Thereafter B. Thereby
    C. Furthermore D. Still
58. A. given B. regarding
    C. in spite of D. speaking of
59. A. parse B. parsed
    C. parsing D. to parse
60. A. potently B. absolutely
    C. potentially D. epidemiologically

Part IV Reading Comprehension (30%)

Directions: *In this part, there are six passages, each of which is followed by five questions. For each question, there are four possible answers marked A, B, C, and D. Choose the best answer and mark the letter of your choice on the* **ANSWER SHEET**.

Passage One

If you're reading this article, antibiotics have probably saved your life—and not once but several times. A rotten tooth, a knee operation, a brush with pneumonia: any number of minor infections that never turned nasty. You may not remember taking the pills, so unremarkable have these one-time wonder drugs become.

Modern medicine relies on antibiotics—not just to cure diseases, but to augment the success of surgery, childbirth and cancer treatments. Yet now health authorities are warning, in uncharacteristically apocalyptic terms, that the era of antibiotics is about to end. In some ways, it has been this way ever since antibiotics became widely available in the 1940s, because bacteria are continually evolving to resist the drugs. But in the past we've always developed new ones that killed them again.

Not this time. Infections that once succumbed to everyday antibiotics now require last-resort drugs with unpleasant side effects. Others have become so difficult to treat that they kill some 25,000 Europeans yearly. And some bacteria now resist every known antibiotic.

Regular readers will know why: *New Scientist* has reported warnings about this for years. We have misused antibiotics appallingly, handing them out to humans like medicinal candy and feeding them to livestock by the tonne, mostly not for health reasons but to make meat cheaper. Now antibiotic-resistant bacteria can be found all over the world—not just in medical facilities, but everywhere from muddy puddles in India to the snows of Antarctica.

How did we reach this point without viable successors to today's increasingly ineffectual drugs? The answer lies not in evolution but economics. Over the past 20 years, nearly every major pharmaceutical company has abandoned antibiotics. Companies must make money, and there isn't much in short-term drugs that should be used sparingly. So researchers have discovered promising candidates, but can't reach into the deep pockets needed to develop them.

This can be fixed. As we report this week, regulatory agencies, worried medical bodies and Big Pharma are finally hatching ways to remedy this market failure. Delinking profits from the volume of drug sold (by adjusting patent rights, say, or offering prizes for innovation) has worked for other drugs, and should work for antibiotics—although there may be a worryingly long wait before they reach the market.

One day, though, these will fall to resistance too. Ultimately, we need evolution-proof cures for bacterial infection: treatments that stop bacteria from causing disease, but don't otherwise inconvenience the little blighters. When resisting drugs confers no selective advantage, drugs will stop breeding resistance.

Researchers have a couple of candidates for such treatment. But they fear regulators will drag their feet over such radical approaches. That, too, can be fixed. We must not neglect development of the sustainable medicine we need, the way we have neglected simple antibiotic R & D (Research and Development).

If we do, one day another top doctor will be telling us that the drugs no longer work—and there really will be no help on the way.

61. In the first paragraph, the author is trying to _____.
    A. warn us against the rampant abuse of antibiotics everywhere
    B. suggest a course of action to reduce antibiotic resistance
    C. tell us a time race between human and bacteria
    D. remind us of the universal benefit of antibiotics

62. The warning from health authorities implies that _____.
    A. the pre-antibiotic era will return
    B. the antibiotic crisis is about to repeat
    C. the wonder drugs are a double-edged sword
    D. the development of new antibiotics is too slow

63. The appalling misuse of antibiotics, according to the passage, _____.
    A. has developed resistant bacteria worldwide
    B. has been mainly practiced for health reasons
    C. has been seldom reported as a warning in the world
    D. has been particularly worsened in the developing countries

64. The market failure refers to _____.

A. the inability to develop more powerful antibiotics

B. the existing increasingly ineffectual drugs in the market

C. the poor management of the major pharmaceutical companies

D. the deprived investment in developing new classes of antibiotics

65. During the presentation of the two solutions, the author carries a tone of _____.

A. doubt   B. urgency

C. indifference   D. helplessness

Passage Two

This issue of Science contains announcements for more than 100 different Gorgon Research Conferences, on topics that range from atomic physics to developmental biology—the brainchild（某人的主意）of Neil Gordon of Johns Hopkins University. These week-long meetings are designed to promote intimate, informal discussion of frontier science. Often confined to fewer than 125 attendees, they have traditionally been held in remote places with minimal distractions. Beginning in the early 1960s, I attended the summer Nucleic Acids Gordon Conference in rural New Hampshire, sharing austere（简朴的）dorm facilities in a private boys' school with randomly assigned roommates. As a beginning scientist, I found the question period after each talk especially fascinating, providing valuable insights into the personalities and ways of thinking of many senior scientists whom I had not encountered previously. Back then, there were no cellphones and no Internet, and all of the speakers seemed to stay for the entire week. During the long, session-free afternoons, graduate students mingled freely with professors. Many lifelong friendships were begun, and—as Gordon intended—new scientific collaborations began. Leap forward to today, and every scientist can gain immediate access to a vast store of scientific thought and to millions of other scientists via the Internet. Why, nevertheless, do in-person scientific meetings remain so valuable for a life in science?

Part of the answer is that science works best when there is a deep mutual trust and understanding between the collaborators, which is hard to develop from a distance. But most important is the critical role that face-to-face scientific meetings play in stimulating a random collision of ideas and approaches. The best new science occurs when someone combines the knowledge gained by other scientists in non-obvious way to create a new understanding of how the world works. A successful scientist needs to deeply believe, whatever the problem being tackled, that there is a better way to approach that problem than the path currently being taken. The scientist is then constantly on the alert for new paths to take in his or her work, which is essential for making breakthroughs. Thus, as much as possible, scientific meetings should be designed to expose the attendees to ways of thinking and techniques that are different from the ones that they already know.

66. Assembled at Gordon Research Conference are those who _____.

A. are physicists and biologists   B. just start doing their science

C. stay in the forefront of science   D. are accomplished senior scientists

67. Speaking of the summer Nucleic Acids Gordon Conference, the author thinks highly of _____.

A. the personalities of senior scientists   B. the question period after each talk

C. the austere facilities around   D. the week-long duration

68. It can be inferred from the author that the value of the in-person scientific conferences _____.

A. does not change with times

B. can be explored online exclusively

C. lies in exchanging the advances in life science

D. is questioned in establishing a vast store of ideas

69. The author believes that the face-to-face scientific conferences can help the attendees better _____.

A. understand what making a breakthrough means to them

B. expose themselves to novel ideas and new approaches

C. foster the passion for doing science

D. tackle the same problem in science

70. What would the author most probably talk about in the following paragraph?

A. How to explore scientific collaborations
B. How to make scientific breakthroughs

C. How to design scientific meetings
D. How to think like a genius

Passage Three

Back in 1896, the Swedish scientist Svante Arrhenius realized that by burning coal we were adding carbon dioxide to the air, and that this would warm the Earth. But he mentioned the issue only in passing（顺便地）, for his calculations suggested it would not become a problem for thousands of years. Others thought that the oceans would soak up any extra CO_2, so there was nothing much to worry about.

That this latter argument has persisted to this day in some quarters highlights our species' propensity（倾向）to underestimate the scale of our impact on the planet. Even the Earth's vast oceans cannot suck up CO_2 as quickly as we can produce it, and we now know the stored CO_2 is acidifying the oceans, a problem in itself.

Now a handful of researchers are warning that energy sources we normally think of as innocuous could affect the planet's climate too. If we start to extract immense amounts of power from the wind, for instance, it will have an impact on how warm water move around the planet, and thus on temperatures and rainfall.

Just to be clear, no one is suggesting we should stop building wind farms on the basis of this risk. Aside from the huge uncertainties about the climatic effects of extracting power from the wind, our present and near-term usage is far too tiny to make any difference. For the moment, any negative consequences on the climate are massively outweighed by the effects of pumping out ever more CO_2. That poses by far the greater environmental threat; weaning ourselves off fossil fuels should remain in the priority.

Even so, now it is the time to start thinking about the long-term effects of the alternative energy sources we are turning to. Those who have already started to look at these issues report weary, indifferent or even hostile reactions to their work.

That's understandable, but disappointing. These effects may be inconsequential, in which case all that will have been wasted is some research time that may well yield interesting insights anyway. Or they may turn out to be sharply negative, in which case the more notice we have, the better. It would be unfortunate to put it mildly, to spend countless trillions replacing fossil-fuel energy infrastructure（基础设施）only to discover that its successor（替代物）is also more damaging that it need be.

These climatic effects may even be beneficial. The first, tentative models suggest that extracting large amounts of energy from high-altitude het streams would cool the planet, counteracting the effects of rising greenhouse gases. It might even be possible to build an energy infrastructure that gives us a degree of control over the weather, turning off wind turbines here, capturing more of the sun's energy there.

We may also need to rethink our long-term research priorities. The sun is ultimately the only source of energy that doesn't end up altering the planet's energy balance. So the best bet might be to invest heavily in improving solar technology and energy storage—rather than in efforts to harness, say, nuclear fusion.

71. In the first two paragraphs, the author is trying to draw our attention to _____.

A. the escalating scale of the global warming

B. the division of scientists over the issue of global warming

C. the reasons for us to worry about extra CO_2 for the oceans

D. the human tendency to underestimate the harmful effects on the planet

72. The author's illustration of wind-power extraction reflects _____.

　A. the priority of protecting the environment

　B. the same human propensity as mentioned previously

　C. the best strategy of reducing the environment threat

　D. the definite huge uncertainties about the climatic effects

73. The author argues that it would be unfortunate to replace fossil fuels only to find out that _____.

　A. the successors are also damaging

　B. the countless trillions spent are wasted

　C. the alternative energy sources don't work

　D. the research invites indifferent or even hostile reactions

74. According to the author, the best strategy is _____.

　A. to counteract the effects of rising greenhouse gases

　B. to develop a degree of control over the weather

　C. to extract large amounts of energy from wind

　D. to explore solar energy and its storage

75. It can be concluded from the passage that we need to take the long view on _____.

　A. human existence on the planet　　　　B. humanity's energy supplies

　C. our environmental threats　　　　　　D. our tendency to myopia

Passage Four

It is a well-known problem: A junior research group leader must somehow compete against the seniors, who have larger laboratories, good funding, and clout（影响）with the journals. Furthermore, in the normal grant system, preliminary data requirements make it hard to start new directions in research. Beginning scientists must build on their postdoctoral work, which forces them to continue along already-trodden paths. Once a laboratory had been established, it is reasonable for the reviewers of competitive grant applications to look for evidence of an investigator's likely success in the form of "preliminary results". But beginning group leaders should be judged only by their demonstrated excellence and their creativity in finding new directions. Such a change would greatly stimulate innovation.

I experienced the advantages of such a system 20 years ago, when moving to Germany from a postdoctoral position in the United States. A hierarchical system（等级系统）that emphasized seniority was rampant in Europe, and independent research position for younger scientists were few, and I was lucky in joining the European Molecular Biology Laboratory (EMBL) in Heidelberg, which was exploring alternative ways to organize science, with the aim of promoting innovation and research excellence.

The EMBL had created a group leader system in which, apart from a few senior scientists to provide some stability, new researchers were directly funded for up to 9 years to do as they pleased, before being required to move on to a senior job elsewhere. This model was a success in large part because this type of funding encouraged a focus on innovation, but also because it provided a separate funding stream in Europe for starting scientists. The EMBL was not alone in this endeavor, as analogous thinking was beginning to take hold at other European institutions and funding agencies. But in 2007, the European system moved an important step further with the introduction of the European Research Council (ERC). The ERC currently runs a pan-European competition that in 2012 funded 536 proposals after receiving more than 4,700 applications from beginning group leaders, each for 5 years for as much as 1.5 million euros per year. This grant program is specifically targeted at providing additional opportunities for young investigators who are "making the transition from working under a supervisor to being independent researchers in their own right." A crucial aspect of the ERC is that the reviewing criteria specifically focus on novelty, interdisciplinary, and high-risk/high-gain research. The ERC runs other competitions to fund established investigators.

76. When it comes to the well-known problem for beginning scientists, what concerns the author is _____.
    A. how to facilitate their creativity
    B. how to motivate them to do science
    C. how to judge their grant applications fairly
    D. how to help them establish their own laboratories

77. To stimulate innovation, the author argues that the current grant system should focus on _____.
    A. the excellence and creativity in exploring new directions
    B. the evidence-based preliminary results for grant application
    C. fair competition between the novel scientists and their seniors
    D. a deep commitment to postdoctoral research on the part of beginning scientists

78. From his personal experience in Germany, the author is trying to tell us that he _____.
    A. realized the universal seniority of the hierarchical grant system
    B. was lucky enough to switch to molecular biology
    C. was a victim of the current grant system
    D. benefited from the system he advocates

79. The funding model created by the EMBL was intended _____.
    A. to ensure the stability of doing science
    B. to place a focus on doing basic sciences
    C. to encourage starting scientists to be innovative
    D. to provide senior positions for qualified scientists

80. Under the grant program of the ERC, starting scientists _____.
    A. are highly recognized by their innovations and discoveries
    B. work as an interdisciplinary team without exception
    C. are independent doing innovative science
    D. gather from different parts of the world

Passage Five

In 2007, surgeons in Aalst, Belgium, were taken aback when part of a surgical robot's arm broke off inside a patient with prostate cancer. The fracture bent the da Vinci robot's instrument so badly that it could not be removed through the original keyhole incision. That meant the urologists had to enlarge the wound to get the instrument out.

Today more than 2,500 of the $1.7 million da Vinci robots are at work in hospitals worldwide, taking part in nearly 1.5 million operations in the past decade. Most patients go home with smaller scars, and the firm that makes da Vinci, Intuitive Surgical of Sunnyvale, California, claims post-operative pain and recovery time are also reduced. But reports of adverse events have risen recently, prompting the US Food and Drug Administration (FDA) to survey surgeons about the system in January. Blooming Business reported earlier this month that 10 product liability lawsuits have been filed against da Vinci's makers in the past 14 months.

The lawsuits, which the firm is defending, make for grisly（严重的）reading – they allege, variously, that da Vinci has caused liver spleen punctures during heart surgery, rectal damage during a prostate operation, and a vaginal hernia after a hysterectomy. There are also a number of cases of unintended burns from the robot's cauterizing tools. The FDA's inquiry, says spokeswoman Synim River, aims to "determine if the rise in reports is a true reflection of problems, or simply an increase due to other factors."

Is there cause for concern? "Rates of adverse events or death for da Vinci surgery have not increased over the past several years," says Intuitive Surgical spokeswoman Lauren Burch, who refused to comment on the lawsuits. "The clinical evidence shows that da Vinci is safer than one open surgical alternative in many common procedures," she says.

The robot aims to offer minimally invasive, highly accurate surgery with a human in control at all times. The surgeon handles the instruments on the robot's four arms from a console with a stereoscopic 3D view of the operation, magnified up to 10 times.

"The console has brilliant, unsurpassed 3D vision, unlike laparoscopic systems with 2D screens," says Ben Challacombe, a consult urologist at Guy's and St Thomas' NHS Foundation Trust in London. "It also has fantastic control instruments that filter out hand tremors, whereas long laparoscopic tools, only enhance tremor." As a regular da Vinci user, Challacombe says the legal issues Intuitive Surgical faces are far more likely to be down to incorrect use by surgeons rather than robot faults.

That view is backed by James Breeden, president of the American Congress of Obstetricians and Gynecologists. "Studies show there is an increased complication rate," he says. And some surgeons only get two days' training on da Vinci.

What's more, healthcare providers are pushing the benefits of robot surgery, Breeden says, advertising less pain, lower blood loss and faster recovery. That drives demand beyond the evidence, he believes. There may not even be good data, claims Breeden, showing "that robotic hysterectomy is even as good as, let alone better than, far less costly minimally invasive alternatives".

81. The increasing uses of robotic surgeries worldwide, according to the passage,_____.
    A. reduce significantly malpractice lawsuits thanks to their safety
    B. put surgeons at a high risk of being sued for malpractice
    C. help hit the record of 1.5 million operations every year
    D. are accompanied by a rise in product liability lawsuits

82. The growing number of the lawsuits _____.
    A. leads to an enquiry by the FDA
    B. reflects the real problems with the firm
    C. has much to do with da Vinci with defects
    D. is ascribed to the improper installation of da Vinci

83. From Burch to Challacombe, we can learn that _____.
    A. such advantages of da Vinci as minimal invasion and high accuracy are questionable
    B. the lawsuits do have the real evidence to be taken seriously
    C. the issue concerning the safety of da Vinci does exist
    D. the surgical robot is not problematic but safe

84. As Breeden argues, the problem lies in _____.
    A. the wrong hands of the surgeons without any qualification
    B. the hidden faults within the instruments on the four arms
    C. the surgical benefits exaggerated by the health providers
    D. a lack of sufficient training on the part of surgeons

85. Which of the following can serve as the best title for the passage?
    A. Four Arms Better Than Two?   B. A Revolution in Surgery?
    C. The True Cost of Surgery?   D. Too Good to Be True?

Passage Six

In a poor, inland, gang-infested part of Los Angeles, there is a clinic for people with type 1 diabetes. As part of the country health care system, it serves persons who have fallen through all other safety-net options, the poorest of the poor. Although type 2 diabetes is rampant in this part of town, type 1 diabetes exists as well. Yet these latter individuals generally lack access to any specialty care—a type of treatment they desperately need due to a complexity of dealing with type 1 diabetes in the setting of poverty and psychosocial stress.

The type 1 Clinic meets one morning per week and is staffed by four endocrinology fellows and a diabetologist, often me, I have the unique perspective of working part of the time in a county setting and the other part of the time in a clinic for people with health insurance, in Beverly Hills. I know what is possible in the treatment of type 1 diabetes. East Los Angeles teaches me what happens when access to care is not available. Most of our patients, in their 20s and 30s and 40s, already have complications of their diabetes: many near end stage. Concepts about maintaining near–normal blood glucose levels often miss their mark- lack of education or money or motivation or factors I can't even imagine make the necessity of a patient acting as his or her own exogenous pancreas nearly impossible, especially when there are acute consequences to hypoglycemia and few to moderate hyperglycemia.

Historically, in spite of these barriers, we persisted and thought we made a difference. Often, teaching simple carbohydrate counting or switching therapy to long-acting insulin improved patients' control and their quality of life. The fellows felt they made a positive impact in the health of their patients. Driving home I would be encouraged by what we had accomplished, although saddened by the severity of the complications suffered by many of our patients.

Yet everything changed with the recession of 2008. In Beverly Hills I heard a lot about the demise of the financial markets. Patients of mine had invested with Bernie Madoff. Some, once billionaires, were millionaires. Personal assistants and housekeepers were laid off; vacation homes were put on the market, parties became less lavish. But all still live in safe, clean homes, wear designer clothes, and eat high-quality food. The landscape is very different for many of my East LA patients. The temporary, part-time jobs they had cobbled together to keep food on the table and pay for housing are gone. I—naively—didn't realize how much worse poverty could get. But now many of our patients are young without food and are becoming homeless. One young man, a college student trying to work his way out of poverty by going to school, lost his job and is living in his car. He is still taking classes but is unable to afford more than a dollar meal from a fast-food restaurant once every day or two. Management of his diabetes involves simply keeping him alive with his erratic, poor eating habits.

86. At the beginning, the author describes the patients with an emphasis on _____.
    A. their financial status
    B. their living in injustice
    C. their specialty care of any kind
    D. their ignorance of type 1 diabetes

87. As a diabetologist working for the type 1 Clinic, the author is quite concerned about those who _____.
    A. misunderstand the concepts on blood glucose maintenance
    B. have no idea about what medical problem they are having
    C. don't care about acting as their own exogenous pancreas
    D. lack access to proper and sufficient clinical care

88. Not until the recession of 2008 did the medical staff _____.
    A. feel proud of their dedication and persistence in clinical practice
    B. know how severe the complications of type 1 diabetes could be
    C. regret about more they could have done for the patients

D. feel a sense of accomplishment in treating the patients

89. As witnessed by the diabetologist during the recession of 2008, many poor patients _____.

    A. developed poor eating habits with the progression of type 1 diabetes

    B. struggled with their survival, let alone with their medical care

    C. became losers in the investment with Bernie Madoff

    D. switched from full-time to part-time jobs

90. Which of the following tones does the passage most probably carry?

    A. Indifference.   B. Sympathy.

    C. Passion.   D. Guilt.

GO TO THE NEXT PAGE FOR PAPER TWO: WRITING.

PAPER TWO

Part V.　Writing (20%)　(50 minutes)

Directions: *In this part, there is an essay in Chinese. Read it carefully and then write a summary of 200 words in English on the **ANSWER SHEET**. Make sure that your summary covers all the major points of the article.*

答题要求
（1）紧扣主题，归纳总结；
（2）涵盖所有重要内容；
（3）避免选择原句进行简单翻译；
（4）无须推演或推论。

环境污染与肺癌

近几十年来，许多国家的流行病学（epidemiology）调查资料都表明，不少传染病的发病率和死亡率在不断下降，而癌症的发病率和死亡率却在不断上升。城市居民癌症和心血管疾病的发病率明显高于农村居民。大量的调查研究表明，癌症等疾病的发病率上升都与环境污染有关。由于环境污染对人体的作用一般具有剂量小、作用时间长等特点，容易被人们所忽视。往往病发之日，尚不知谁是元凶。

环境污染就像邪恶的阴影，悄悄吞噬着人体的健康。肺及呼吸道是一个开放器官，与外界直接接触，外界很多致癌因素（carcinogenic factor）都可以导致肺癌。环境污染就是导致肺癌的一个重要原因。环境污染中最为重要的就是大气污染（air pollution）。许多研究大气污染的学者惊奇地发现，近 50 年来，随着工业和经济的发展，人们生活水平的提高，肺癌的发病率也显著提高，特别是世界经济发达地区的患者成倍地增加。例如，美国的病人数量在 50 年中，男性增加了 18 倍，女性增加了 6 倍，每 4 名癌症死亡病例中，就有 1 名是肺癌患者；每 100 名死亡病人中，有 5 名死于肺癌。就我国情况看，也有明显增加的趋势。从全国恶性肿瘤（malignant tumor）排列顺序来看，肺癌占第 5 位；每 100 名癌症病人中，大约有 8 名患的是肺癌。

肺癌是最常见的恶性肿瘤之一，据 WHO 统计，每年全球估计有 120 万以上新发肺癌病例，死亡约万人。近年来，我国肺癌发病率及死亡率亦不断上升。国外流行病学研究报告，大气污染易诱发肺癌而使死亡率增高。

在公认的大气污染物（air pollutants）中，颗粒物（particulate matter）对健康的危害最大，可增加患肺癌的危险。随着交通的发展、机动车辆的增加、环境的日益破坏，PM2.5 污染越来越严重。研究发现，大气中 PM2.5 在总悬浮颗粒物中的比率逐年增加，沉积在下呼吸道的 96% 颗粒物是 PM2.5。对肺癌死亡率进行分析表明市区大气总悬浮颗粒物（total suspended particulates）与肺癌死亡率增高有一定的相关性。这在世界许多国家都被证实。美国癌症协会收集的 16 年资料，涉及 500,000 名美国人的死亡原因数据，发现空气中的 PM2.5 与总死亡率和肺癌死亡相关。在日本进行的 PM2.5 与疾病关系研究也发现，PM2.5 水平与女性肺癌呈正相关。

THIS IS THE END OF THIS OFFICIAL TEST.

Hi-Fi FATMD Test 1
Answer Keys
（非标准答案，仅供参考）

Part Ⅰ. Listening

1-3: DCA   4-6: ADB   7-9: CAD   10-12: CDA   13-15: ACB   16-18: BDC   19-21: DCB

22-24: BDD   25-27: ACD   28-30: BCA

Part Ⅱ. Vocabulary

31-35: ACBCD   36-40: BABAD   41-45: BDCCD   46-50: ACCAC

Part Ⅲ. Cloze

51-55: BBDAC   56-60: ADACC

Part Ⅳ. Reading Comprehension

61-65: DAADD   66-70: CBABC   71-75: DBADB   76-80:CADCA   81-85: DADDA

86-90: ADBBB

Part Ⅴ. Writing Sample

Environmental Pollution and Lung Cancer

Recent epidemiological studies have revealed a concerning trend: as infectious diseases decline, cancer rates are steadily rising. Urban residents, in particular, suffer higher incidences of cancer and cardiovascular conditions compared to their rural counterparts. Extensive research consistently links this rise in cancer to environmental pollution, a factor often underestimated due to its subtle, long-term effects. Notably, lung cancer is strongly associated with environmental pollution, particularly air pollution. Over the past 50 years, economically developed regions have witnessed a significant increase in lung cancer cases. In the United States, the number of male patients has escalated by 18 times, while females have experienced a six-fold surge. This alarming correlation is supported globally. Particulate matter, especially fine particles measuring 2.5 micrometres or less (PM2.5), represents the most detrimental air pollutant contributing to lung cancer risk. The proportion of PM2.5 within total suspended particulate matter has seen a continuous rise, with 96% of such particles deposited in the lower respiratory tract. Studies have demonstrated a direct correlation between urban areas with high levels of PM2.5 and increased lung cancer mortality rates, further highlighting the urgent need to address and alleviate the detrimental health effects of environmental pollution, with a specific emphasis on lung health.

Tapescript for the Listening Comprehension

Section A

Conversation One (Word count: 168)

Doctor: Mm, your blood pressure is a bit on the high side, Mr. Dean.

Patient: Oh.

Doctor: I'll take it again in a few minutes ... It's gone down a little, but it's still a bit higher than it should be. (1. D) It's important that we control it. Do you understand why it's important to control your blood pressure?

Patient: It can cause a stroke or a heart attack.

Doctor: Yes, that's right. Now, there are a number of options you could consider. So firstly, I'll outline what they are, and then I'll talk about each treatment in turn. OK?

Patient: Fine.

Doctor: In terms of medication, the following options are available. You could consider taking water pills or diuretics（利尿剂）. These flush out excess fluid and salt in your body, which helps to lower blood pressure. (3. A)

Patient: Ah.

Doctor: Another option is taking beta-blockers（beta 阻断剂）. Basically, these block the effects of adrenalin（肾上腺素）on the heart, reducing the amount of stress to the heart. This means the heart doesn't have to work so hard, and therefore blood pressure is reduced.

Doctor: The other option you could try is adopting a healthy lifestyle plan. (2. C)

Questions 1 to 3 are based on the conversation you've just heard.

1. What's the patient's problem?   D)（主旨概括）
2. Which of the following DOESN'T the doctor advise?   C)（具体细节）
3. What is the effect of diuretics, according to the doctor?   A)（判断推理）

Conversation Two (Word count: 134)

M: Your doctor says that you have a cough. Could you please tell me more about it and about any other symptoms you may have?

W: Well, I've had this cough for about two months now, and sometimes I feel short of breath, particularly in the morning. (5. D)

M: Could you tell me if you bring up any sputum when you cough?

W: Yes, sometimes I do in the morning, but I think that's because I smoke, although I am trying to cut down. Also, I wheeze, particularly when I'm at work, and I think that's due to the air conditioning.

M: You seem to have two concerns. First, you want to stop smoking, and I am sure that this is important for your health. Second, you are worried about your work. How do you think that I can help?

Questions 4 to 6 are based on the conversation you've just heard.

4. What is the probable relationship between the two speakers?   A)（判断推理）
5. What problem brings the woman to the man?   D)（具体细节）
6. What does the man want to learn from the woman?   B)（推断推理）

Conversation Three (Word count: 137)

M: Dr. Brook, I just don't know what's wrong with me. I always feel tired and rundown. (7.C) My wife finally persuaded me to visit you to find out what the trouble is.

W: Looking at your case history, I see that you had pneumonia four years ago and that you also had a minor operation last year. Did you have any long-term after-effects?

M: Well, I don't remember so.

W: For instance, how long did you stay at home each time?

M: Just a couple of days. (8. A) But about six months ago, I was home for about two weeks with a cold or something.

W: Did you see a doctor at that time, or did you just stay at home?

M: No, I didn't see a doctor. The symptoms were about the same as this time. When I began to feel better, I returned to work. (9. D)

Questions 7 to 9 are based on the conversation you've just heard.

7. Why is the patient seeing the doctor?　　　　　　　　　　　C)（主旨概括）

8. How long did the man stay at home after he had pneumonia?　A)（具体细节）

9. When did the man return to work the last time he was sick?　D)（具体细节）

Conversation Four (Word count: 84)

Doctor: Hello, Miss Lennox. What can I do for you?

Patient: The antibiotics you prescribed haven't cleared up my chest infection.

Doctor: Right. Did you complete the course?

Patient: Yes, I did.

Doctor: And do you feel any better after taking them?

Patient: No. They've had absolutely no effect, apart from giving me thrush（皮疹）and leaving me feeling completely washed out (10. C)

Doctor: Right. I'm sorry to hear that. Sometimes antibiotics may not agree with patients. (12. A) What I'll do is try you with a different antibiotic and see how that goes.

Questions 10 to 12 are based on the conversation you've just heard.

10. What's the problem with the patient?　　　　　　　　　　C)（主旨概括）

11. Which of the following the patient doesn't complain of?　　D)（具体细节）

12. How does the doctor explain the problem?　　　　　　　　A)（具体细节）

Conversation Five (Word count: 177)

James: So, I've got AIDS?

Doctor: Well, you're HIV positive, (13. A) which means that you have been exposed to HIV virus, which causes AIDS. It can take a long time to develop into AIDS, but from the symptoms we observed on your last visit, there is a possibility that it's happening already.

James: Right.

Doctor: Can you tell me how you're feeling, James?

James: I'm really scared. One of my friends died of AIDS two years ago (14. C)

Doctor: It's only natural that you feel scared.

James: So, can it be treated?

Doctor: There are drugs that can help. Would you like me to tell you about them?

James: Not right now, doctor. I'm not able to take much in at the moment.

Doctor: I can understand that. We can go through it at your next appointment.

James: OK. What are my chances?

Doctor: I realize how difficult it must be for you to ask that question. I can't really say at this point, but we'll do everything we can. Do you have a friend or relative you can talk to about this?

James: I'm really close to my sister. (15. B)

Doctor: That's good.

Questions 13 to 15 are based on the conversation you've just heard.

13. What is James's problem?　　　　　　　　　　　　　　　A)（主旨概括）

14. Why is James scared?　　　　　　　　　　　　　　　　C)（具体细节）

15. Which of the following people is the closest to James?　　B)（判断推理）

Section B

Passage One (Word count: 106)

Hello, everyone. In the last session, we have discussed how different cultures perceive illness, care and treatment in different ways. From that discussion, we have learned the importance of cross-cultural communication in medical treatment and services. In today's class, we'll mainly focus on the problem of language in such situations. (17. D)

Language is foremost among problems in cross-cultural communication. Even when the patient is familiar with the language of the majority culture, there are nuances, metaphors, idiomatic expressions and non-verbal cues that can cause misunderstanding or confusion for non-native speakers. Misunderstanding can threaten the doctor-patient relationship and also have serious implications for the patient's care. (16. C)

Questions 16 to 18 are based on the passage you've just heard.

16. Who might be the audience of the talk?　　　　　　　　　　　　　　　B）（判断推理）
17. What might be the best title for the woman's talk?　　　　　　　　　　D）（主旨概括）
18. According to the speaker, what might be the effects of misunderstanding?　C）（具体细节）

Passage Two (Word count: 170)

Exercise is good for health, but some kinds of exercise may be better than others. Running, for example, may help prevent heart disease and other health problems. Running may also help you live longer.

It is not important how far you run or how fast or even how often you run. But it is important to "just do it." (19. D)

Recently, researchers have studied over 55,000 adults. About 1/4 of them reported running regularly. The study found these runners were considerably less likely than non-runners to die of any form of disease, including heart disease. In fact, the runners lived, on average, 3 years longer than the non-runners. This study lasted 15 years. During that time, more than 3,400 of all the subjects died. About 1,200 of the deaths were linked to heart disease, a heart attack or stroke. (20. C)

Dr. D.C. Lee says, "Compared to non-runners, runners showed a much lower risk of dying from some diseases." "Compared to non-runners, runners showed 30 per cent lower risk of death by any causes, (21. B) including heart attack, stroke or cancer.

Questions 19 to 21 are based on the passage you've just heard.

19. What is this passage mainly about?　　　　　　　　　　　　　　　　D）（主旨概括）
20. Among all the subjects of the study, how many died from heart disease?　C）（具体细节）
21. What is true about the risk of death of runners compared with non-runners?　B）（判断推理）

Passage Three (Word count: 106)

Thanks, Dr. Kapinsky. I'm going to talk today about some of the issues surrounding the history-taking process of older patients. Enlow talked about the fear felt by a great many older people of losing their independence (22. B), which is sometimes greater than the illness itself. We need, therefore, to look at the ADL, the activities of daily living (23. D) used to assess the level of independence in an older patient within their environment. (24. D) You can also gauge the patient's own perception of their independence using this tool. Has anyone heard of BATTED-B-A-T-T-E-D?

Questions 22 to 24 are based on the passage you've just heard.

22. What are many aged people afraid of?　　　　　　　　　　　　　　　B）（判断推理）
23. What is ADL according to the passage?　　　　　　　　　　　　　　D）（具体细节）
24. What might be the speaker's major concern in his talk?　　　　　　　D）（主旨概括）

Passage Four (Word count: 132)

So, moving on to the past medical history. Patients of all age groups have problems retrieving information about their PMH (past medical history) and may need a little coaxing. (25. A) You can begin with an open question but move on to closed questions; after all, you are looking for information that is directly related to the presenting complaint. However, be careful that you're not interrogating the patient either and bombarding them with questions (26. C); give them time to reflect before going on to the next component.

Start by asking about patients' past illnesses. More recent illnesses are OK, but patients are often vague about those that took place further back unless there is some kind of landmark (27. A)—a particular stage in their life or a traumatic event, a death in the family, for example.

Questions 25 to 27 are based on the passage you've just heard.

25. What is the major topic of the talk?　　　　　　　　　　　　　A)（主旨概括）

26. Which of the following should a doctor avoid when asking for medical history?　C)（具体细节）

27. What might be the problem with patients recalling their past illnesses?　　A)（判断推理）

Passage Five (Word count: 132)

Well, ladies and Gentlemen. Now that we have had a ward round, (28. B) let me brief you on the case history of Mr. Wildgoose, a retired bus driver at the age of 61. He was unwell and in bed with a cough and general malaise when he called in his general practitioner (GP). A lower respiratory tract infection was diagnosed, and erythromycin was prescribed. Two days later, at a second home visit, he was found to be a little breathless and complaining that he felt worse. He was advised to drink plenty and to continue with his antibiotic. Another 2 days passed, and the general practitioner returned to find the patient barely rousable（几乎起不了床）and breathless at rest. Emergency admission to hospital was arranged on the grounds of severe chest infection. (29. C)

Questions 28 to 30 are based on the passage you've just heard.

28. At what time was this talk probably given?　　　　　　　　　　B)（判断推理）

29. Why was the patient admitted to the emergency room?　　　　　C)（具体细节）

30. When was the patient hospitalized?　　　　　　　　　　　　　A)（具体细节）

Hi-Fi FATMD Test 2

国家医学考试中心标准答题卡

书 面 表 达　　　　　　请用黑色签字笔在答题区域内作答，超出黑色边框区域的答案无效！

15

20

25

30

LT–1/8R 2013B002B

Hi-Fi FATMD Test 2

PAPER ONE

Part Ⅰ　Listening Comprehension (30%)

Section A

Directions: *In this section, you will hear five conversations. At the end of each conversation, you will hear three questions about the conversation. The question will be read only once. After you hear the question, read the four choices marked A, B, C, and D. Choose the best answer and mark the letter of your choice on the* **ANSWER SHEET**.

Sample Answer
A　B　●　D

Listen to the following example.

You will hear:

　　W: Can you tell me about yourself, please?

　　M: Sure, my name's Harry, 18 years old, currently studying biology and chemistry at school. As you are aware, I hope to pursue a career in medicine.

　　W: Harry, why do you want to be a doctor?

　　M: Well, everyone in my family is a doctor, so I think I can follow on nicely. (2. A)

　　W: Apart from treating patients, what do you think being a doctor is going to require?

　　M: Well, you also need to be academic and have to be an excellent communicator (3. B)with your team and the patients.

　　Questions number 1 to 3 are based on the conversation you have just heard.

　　Question No. 1: What are the two speakers talking about?

You will read:

1.　A. Switching to biology and chemistry.

　　B. Choosing to be a family physician.

　　C. Going to college.

　　D. **Being a doctor.**

　　The correct answer is D. Mark the right answer on the **ANSWER SHEET** *as indicated below:*

1. A　B　C　●

　　Question No. 2: Why does Harry choose to be a doctor?

You will read:

2.　A. **Because of his family influence.**

　　B. Because of the fact that he's young.

　　C. Because of the practical skills he has.

　　D. Because of his love for biology and chemistry.

　　The correct answer is A. Mark the right answer on the **ANSWER SHEET** *as indicated below:*

2. ●　B　C　D

Question No. 3: What is mentioned by Harry as one of the requirements for a doctor?
You will read:
3.　A. A strong sense of responsibility.
　　B. **Good communicative skills.**
　　C. Excellent health.
　　D. Great patience.
The correct answer is B. Mark the right answer on the **ANSWER SHEET** *as indicated below:*

3. A　●　C　D

Now let's begin with Conversation One.
Conversation One
1.　A. Doing a physical checkup for the patient.　B. Doing sit-ups for exercise.
　　C. Practicing deep breathing.　D. Performing hypnotism on the patient.
2.　A. Nineteen.　B. Ninety-nine.
　　C. Nine.　D. Ninety.
3.　A. Ask the patient to have further examinations.
　　B. Ask the patient to do push-ups.
　　C. Take the patient's blood pressure again.
　　D. Ask the patient to do deep breathing.

Conversation Two
4.　A. He can't find the key to his office.　B. He needs to find a substitute.
　　C. He needs to speak with his professor.　D. He is sick.
5.　A. He can't talk due to a throat infection.　B. His wildlife videotape player is broken.
　　C. There are American rodents in his bedroom.　D. He has lost his materials.
6.　A. Grade the class papers.　B. Make a movie.
　　C. Show a movie.　D. Help him find the class.

Conversation Three
7.　A. Last week.　B. Four hours ago.
　　C. Yesterday.　D. Six days ago.
8.　A. She need to take more exercise.　B. Her uncle's health has not improved.
　　C. She can't understand the doctor.　D. Her ankle is swollen.
9.　A. To sit at home for four days.　B. To take four tablets a day.
　　C. To sit for four hours a day with her leg raised.　D. To ask her uncle to raise her four times a day.

Conversation Four
10.　A. The woman's toothache.　B. Teeth made of plastics.
　　C. Tooth transplant.　D. The medical school in New York.
11.　A. The woman prefers filling the bad tooth to taking it out.
　　B. They both hate to have a tooth filled.
　　C. They both would rather have a tooth filled.
　　D. The man prefers to have the bad tooth filled rather than pulled.
12.　A. Nobody was doing anything to prevent tooth trouble.
　　B. The filling stopped teeth from falling out.
　　C. Dentists put animals on the moon.
　　D. Doctors can transplant hearts.

Conversation Five

13. A. The diseases of willow trees.
    C. The possibility of tree communication.
    B. The smell of willow.
    D. The need to preserve the wilderness.

14. A. Suspicious.
    C. Interested.
    B. Hostile.
    D. Unconcerned.

15. A. They began to speak.
    C. They became infected.
    B. They made a strange smell.
    D. They cured themselves.

Section B

Directions: *In this section, you will hear five passages. At the end of each passage, you will hear three questions about the passage. The question will be spoken only once. After you hear the question, read the four possible answers labeled A, B, C, and D. Choose the best answer and mark the letter of your choice on the* **ANSWER SHEET.**

Sample Answer
A B ● D

Passage One

16. A. Impact of inadequate sleep on students' academic performance.
    B. Why students have inadequate sleep.
    C. How much sleep students should have.
    D. Insufficient sleep and attention problem.

17. A. Monitor students' sleep patterns.
    C. Record students' weekly performance.
    B. Help students concentrate in class.
    D. Ask students to complete a sleep report.

18. A. Declining health.
    C. Loss of motivation.
    B. Lack of attention.
    D. Improper behaviour.

Passage Two

19. A. The harmful effects of obesity.
    C. Obesity in the world.
    B. The incidence of birth defects.
    D. Unhealthy lifestyle.

20. A. On the decline.
    C. Serious enough to be fatal.
    B. Likely to go unnoticed.
    D. Caused by an obese mother.

21. A. 20 million.
    C. 200 million.
    B. 40 million.
    D. 400 million.

Passage Three

22. A. Historical accounts of drug usage in the West.
    B. Recipes for producing medicines.
    C. Medical techniques.
    D. Records of patients in the West.

23. A. The age of the books.
    C. The emphasis on simplicity and practicality.
    B. The people who were helped by the books.
    D. The technical superiority of the books.

24. A. Roche.
    C. Pfizer.
    B. Johnson.
    D. Merck.

Passage Four

25. A. Nitrogen's role in the atmosphere.
    C. The noble gasses.
    B. Safety and liquid Nitrogen.
    D. Reactions in very cool substances.

26. A. To explain the chemistry of the atmosphere.
    B. To facilitate a quiz.

C. To break a pencil.   D. To fill up a balloon.

27. A. The desk was cold.   B. The tongs crushed it.

    C. It was frozen solid.   D. The professor broke it with his hand.

Passage Five

28. A. Stress factors.   B. Working too long.

    C. TV watching.   D. The general American culture.

29. A. A third.   B. Almost two thirds.

    C. More than two thirds.   D. Almost half.

30. A. Eight hours.

    B. Seven hours.

    C. Six hours.

    D. Seven hours each week night and more on weekends.

Part Ⅱ   Vocabulary (10%)

Section A

Directions: *In this section, all the sentences are incomplete. Beneath each of them are given four words or phrases, marked A, B, C, and D. Choose the word or phrase that best completes the sentence. Then, mark the letter of your choice on the* **ANSWER SHEET***.*

31. There was no _____ but to close the road until February.

    A. dilemma   B. denying

    C. alternative   D. doubt

32. I _____ when I heard that my grandfather had died.

    A. fell apart   B. fell away

    C. fell out   D. fell back

33. I'm _____ passing a new law that helps poor children get better medicine.

    A. taking advantage of   B. standing up for

    C. looking up to   D. taking hold of

34. In front of the platform, the students were talking with the professor over the quizzes of their _____ subjects.

    A. compulsory   B. compulsive

    C. alternative   D. predominant

35. The tutor tells the undergraduates that one can acquire _____ in a foreign language through more practice.

    A. proficiency   B. efficiency

    C. efficacy   D. frequency

36. The teacher explained the new lesson _____ to the students.

    A. at random   B. at a loss

    C. at length   D. at hand

37. I shall _____ the loss of my reading-glasses in newspaper with a reward for the finder.

    A. advertise   B. inform

    C. announce   D. publish

38. The poor nutrition in the early stages of infancy can _____ adult growth.

    A. degenerate   B. deteriorate

C. boost   D. retard

39. She had a terrible accident, but _____ she wasn't killed.

    A. at all events   B. in the long run

    C. at large   D. in vain

40. His weak chest _____ him to winter illness.

    A. predicts   B. preoccupies

    C. prevails   D. predisposes

Section B

Directions: *Each of the following sentences has a word or phrase underlined. Beneath each sentence there are four words or phrases marked A, B, C, and D. Choose the word or phrase which can best keep the meaning of the original sentence if it is substituted for the underlined part. Mark the letter of your choice on the* **ANSWER SHEET**.

41. The company was losing money, so they had to lay off some of its employees for three months.

    A. owe   B. dismiss

    C. recruit   D. summon

42. The North American states agreed to sign the agreement of economical and military union in Ottawa.

    A. convention   B. conviction

    C. contradiction   D. confrontation

43. The statue would be perfect but for a few small defects in its base.

    A. faults   B. weaknesses

    C. flaws   D. errors

44. When he finally emerged from the cave after thirty days, John was startlingly pale.

    A. amazingly   B. astonishingly

    C. uniquely   D. dramatically

45. If you want to set up a company, you must comply with the regulations laid down by the authorities.

    A. abide by   B. work out

    C. check out   D. succumb to

46. The school master applauded the girl's bravery in his opening speech.

    A. praised   B. appraised

    C. cheered   D. clapped

47. The local government leaders are making every effort to tackle the problem of poverty.

    A. abolish   B. address

    C. extinguish   D. encounter

48. This report would be intelligible only to an expert in computing.

    A. intelligent   B. comprehensive

    C. competent   D. comprehensible

49. Reading a book and listening to music simultaneously seems to be no problem for them.

    A. intermittently   B. constantly

    C. concurrently   D. continuously

50. He was given a laptop computer in acknowledgement of his work for the company.

    A. accomplishment   B. recognition

    C. apprehension   D. commitment

Part Ⅲ　Cloze (10%)

Directions: *In this section, there is a passage with ten numbered blanks. For each blank, there are four choices marked A, B, C, and D on the right side. Choose the best answer and mark the letter of your choice on the* **ANSWER SHEET**.

In Mr. Allen's high school class, all the students have to "get married". However, the wedding ceremonies are not real ones but　51　. These mock ceremonies sometimes become so　52　that the loud laughter drowns out the voice of the "minister". Even the two students getting married often begin to giggle.

The teacher, Mr. Allen, believes that marriage is a difficult and serious business. He wants young people to understand that there are many changes that　53　take place after marriage. He believes that the need for these psychological and financial　54　should be understood before people marry.

Mr. Allen doesn't only introduce his students to major problems　55　in marriage such as illness or unemployment. He also exposes them to nitty-gritty problems they will face every day. He wants to introduce young people to all the trials and　56　that can strain a marriage to the breaking point. He even　57　his students with the problems of divorce and the fact that divorced men must pay child support money for their children and sometimes pay monthly alimony to their wives.

It has been upsetting for some of the students to see the problems that a married couple often faces.　58　they took the course, they had not worried much about the problems of marriage. However, both students and parents feel that Mr. Allen's course is valuable and have　59　the course publicly. Their statements and letters supporting the class have,　60　the school to offer the course again.

51. A. duplications　　B. imitations
　　C. assumptions　　D. fantasies

52. A. noisy　　B. artificial
　　C. graceful　　D. real

53. A. might　　B. would
　　C. must　　D. need

54. A. issues　　B. adjustments
　　C. matters　　D. expectancies

55. A. to face　　B. facing
　　C. having faced　　D. faced

56. A. tribulations　　B. errors
　　C. triumphs　　D. verdicts

57. A. informs　　B. concerns
　　C. triumphs　　D. associates

58. A. Until　　B. Before
　　C. After　　D. As

59. A. taken　　B. suggested
　　C. endorsed　　D. reproached

60. A. confirmed　　B. convinced
　　C. compromised　　D. conceived

Part Ⅳ　Reading Comprehension (30%)

Directions: *In this part there are six passages, each of which is followed by five questions. For each question there are four possible answers marked A, B, C, and D. Choose the best answer and mark the letter of your choice on the* **ANSWER SHEET**.

Passage One

Why do people always want to get up and dance when they hear music? The usual explanation is that there is something embedded in every culture—that dancing is a "cultural universal". A researcher in Manchester thinks the impulse may be even more deeply rooted than that. He says it may be a reflex reaction.

Neil Todd, a psychologist at the University of Manchester, told the BA that he first got an inkling that biology was the key after watching people dance to deafeningly loud music. "There is a compulsion about it," he says. He reckoned there might be a more direct, biological, explanation for the desire to dance, so he started to look at the inner ear.

The human ear has two main functions: hearing and maintaining balance. The standard view is that these tasks are segregated so that organs for balance, for instance, do not have an acoustic function. But Todd says animal studies have shown that the sacculus, which is part of the balance—regulating vestibular system, has retained some sensitivity to sound. The sacculus is especially sensitive to extremely loud noise, above 70 decibels.

"There's no doubt that in a contemporary dance environment, the sacculus will be stimulated," says Todd. The average rave, he says, blares music at a painful 110 to 140 decibels. But no one really knows what an acoustically stimulated sacculus does.

Todd speculates that listening to extremely loud music is a form of "vestibular self-stimulation": it gives a heightened sensation of motion. "We don't know exactly why it causes pleasure," he says. "But we know that people go to extraordinary lengths to get it." He lists bungee jumping, playing on swings or even rocking to and fro in a rocking chair as other examples of pursuits designed to stimulate the sacculus.

The same pulsing that makes us feel as though we are moving may make us get up and dance as well, says Todd. Loud music sends signals to the inner ear which may prompt reflex movement. "The typical pulse rate of dance music is around the rate of locomotion," he says. "It's quite possible you're triggering a spinal reflex."

61. The passage begins with _____.
   A. a new explanation of music
   B. a cultural universal question
   C. a common psychological abnormality
   D. a deep insight into human physical movements

62. What intrigued Todd was _____.
   A. human instinct reflexes
   B. people's biological heritages
   C. people's compulsion about loud music
   D. the damages loud music wrecks on human hearing

63. Todd's biological explanation for the desire to dance refers to _____.
   A. the mechanism of hearing sounds
   B. the response evoked from the sacculus
   C. the two main functions performed by the human ear
   D. the segregation of the hearing and balance maintaining function

64. When the sacculus is acoustically stimulated, according to Todd, _____.
   A. functional balance will be maintained in the ear
   B. pleasure will be aroused
   C. decibels will shoot up
   D. hearing will occur

65. What is the passage mainly about?
   A. The human ear does more than hearing than expected.
   B. Dancing is capable of heightening the sensation of hearing.
   C. Loud music stimulates the inner ear and generates the urge to dance.
   D. The human inner ear does more to help hear than to help maintain balance.

Passage Two

Have you switched off your computer? How about your television? Your video? Your CD player? And even your coffee percolator? Really switched them off, not just pressed the button on some control panel and left your machine with a telltale bright red light warning you that it is ready to jump back to life at your command?

Because if you haven't, you are one of the guilty people who are helping to pollute the planet. It doesn't matter if you've joined the neighborhood recycling scheme, conscientiously sorted your garbage and avoided driving to work. You still can't sleep easy while just one of those little red lights is glowing in the dark.

The awful truth is that household and office electrical appliances left on stand-by mode are gobbling up energy, even though they are doing absolutely nothing. Some electronic products—such as CD players —can use almost as much energy on stand-by as they do when running. Others may use a lot less, but as your video player spends far more hours on stand-by than playing anything, the wastage soon adds up.

In the US alone, *idle electronic devices* consume enough energy to power cities with the energy needs of Chicago or London — costing consumers around $1 billion a year. Power stations fill the atmosphere with carbon dioxide just to do absolutely nothing.

Thoughtless design is partly responsible for the waste. But manufacturers only get away with designing products that waste energy this way because consumers are not sensitive enough to the issue. Indeed, while recycling has caught the public imagination, reducing waste has attracted much less attention.

But "source reduction", as the garbage experts like to call the art of not using what you don't need to use, offers enormous potential for reducing waste of all kinds. With a little intelligent shopping, you can cut waste long before you reach the end of the chain.

Packaging remains the big villain. One of the hidden consequences of buying products grown or made all around the world, rather than produced locally, is the huge amount of packaging needed to transport them safely. In the US, a third of the solid waste collected from city homes is packaging. To help cut the waste and encourage intelligent manufacturers the simplest trick is to look for ultra-light packaging.

The same arguments apply to the very light but strong plastic bottles that are replacing heavier glass alternatives, thin-walled aluminum cans, and cartons made of composites that wrap up anything drinkable in an ultra-light package.

There are hundreds of other tricks you can discuss with colleagues while gathering around the proverbial water cooler—filling up, naturally, your own mug rather than a disposable plastic cup. But you don't need to go as far as one website which tells you how to give your friends unwrapped Christmas presents. There are limits to source correctness.

66. From the first two paragraphs, the author implies that _____.
    A. hitechnic has made life easy everywhere
    B. nobody seems to be innocent in polluting the planet
    C. recycling can potentially control environmental deterioration
    D. everybody is joining the global battle against pollution in one way or another

67. The waste caused by household and office electrical appliances on stand-by mode seems to _____.
    A. be a long-standing indoor problem   B. cause nothing but trouble
    C. get exaggerated   D. go unnoticed

68. By *idle electronic devices*, the author means those appliances _____.
    A. left on stand-by mode
    B. filling the atmosphere with carbon dioxide
    C. used by those who are not energy-conscious
    D. used by those whose words speak louder than actions

69. Ultra-light packaging _____.
    A. is expected to reduce American waste by one-third

B. is an illustration of what is called "source reduction"

C. can make both manufacturers and consumers intelligent

D. is a villain of what the garbage experts call "source reduction"

70. The conclusion the author is trying to draw is that _____.

A. one person cannot win the battle against pollution

B. anybody can pick up tricks of environmental protection on the web

C. nobody can be absolutely right in all the tricks of environmental protection

D. anybody can present or learn a trick of cutting down what is not needed

Passage Three

You can have too much of a good thing, it seems—at least when it comes to physiotherapy after a stroke. Many doctors believe that it is the key to recovery: exercising a partially paralyzed limb can help the brain "rewire" itself and replace neural connections destroyed by a clot in the brain.

But the latest animal experiments suggest that too much exercise too soon after a brain injury can make the damage worse. "It's something that clinicians are not aware of," says Timothy Schallert of the University at Austin, who led the research.

In some trials, stroke victims asked to put their good arm in a sling—to force them to use their partially paralyzed limb—had made much better recoveries than those who used their good arm. But these patients were treated many months after their strokes. Earlier intervention, Schallert reasoned, should lead to even more dramatic improvements.

To test this theory, Schallert and his colleagues placed tiny casts on the good forelimbs of rats for two weeks immediately after they were given a small brain injury that partially paralyzed one forelimb. Several weeks later, the researchers were astonished to find that brain tissue surrounding the original injury had also died. "The size of the injury doubled. It's a very dramatic effect." says Schallert.

Brain-injured rats that were not forced to overuse their partially paralyzed limbs showed no similar damage, and the casts did not cause a dramatic loss of brain tissue in animals that had not already suffered minor brain damage. In subsequent experiments, the researchers have found that the critical period for exercise-induced damage in rats is the first week after the initial brain injury.

The spreading brain damage witnessed by Schallert's team was probably caused by the release of glutamate, a neurotransmitter, from brain cells stimulated during limb movement. At high doses, glutamate is toxic even to healthy nerve cells. And Schallert believes that a brain injury makes neighboring cells unusually susceptible to the neurotransmitter's toxic effects.

Randolph Nudo of the University of Texas Health Science Center at Houston, who studies brain injury in primates, agrees that glutamate is the most likely culprit. In experiments with squirrel monkeys suffering from stroke-like damage, Nudo tried beginning rehabilitation within five days of injury. Although the treatment was beneficial in the long run, Nudo noticed an initial worsening of the paralysis that might also have been due to brain damage brought on by exercise.

Schallert stresses that mild exercise is likely to be beneficial however soon it begins. He adds that it is unclear whether human victims of strokes, like brain-injured rats, could make their problems worse by exercising too vigorously, too soon.

Some clinics do encourage patients to begin physiotherapy within a few weeks of suffering a traumatic head injury or stroke, says David Hovda, director of brain injury research at the University of California, Los Angeles. But even if humans do have a similar period of vulnerability to rats, he speculates that it might be possible to use drugs to block the effects of glutamate.

71. Schallert issued a warning to those who _____.
    A. believe in the possibility of rewiring the brain
    B. are ignorant of physiotherapy in the clinic
    C. add exercise to partially paralyzed limbs
    D. are on the verge of a stroke

72. Which of the following is Schallert's hypothesis for his investigation?
    A. Earlier intervention should lead to even more dramatic improvements.
    B. The critical period for brain damage is one week after injury.
    C. A partially paralyzed limb can cause brain damages.
    D. Physiotherapy is the key to brain recovery.

73. The results from Schallert's research _____.
    A. reinforced the significance of physiotherapy after a stroke
    B. indicated the fault with his experiment design
    C. turned out the opposite
    D. verified his hypothesis

74. The results made Schallert's team aware of the fact that _____.
    A. glutamate can have toxic effects on healthy nerve sells
    B. exercise can boost the release of glutamate
    C. glutamate is a neurotransmitter
    D. all of the above

75. Schallert would probably advise clinicians _____.
    A. to administer drugs to block the effects of glutamate
    B. to be watchful of the amount of exercise for stroke victims
    C. to prescribe vigorous exercise to stroke victims one week after injury
    D. to reconsider the significance of physiotherapy to brain damage

Passage Four

Our understanding of cities in anything more than casual terms usually starts with observations of their spatial form and structure at some point or cross-section in time. This is the easiest way to begin, for it is hard to assemble data on how cities change through time, and, in any case, our perceptions often betray us into thinking of spatial structures as being resilient and long lasting. Even where physical change is very rapid, this only has an impact on us when we visit such places infrequently, after years away. Most of our urban theory, whether it emanates from the social sciences or engineering, is structured around the notion that spatial and social structures change slowly, and are sufficiently inert for us to infer reasonable explanations from cross-sectional studies. In recent years, these assumptions have come to be challenged, and in previous editorials I have argued the need for a more temporal emphasis to our theories and models, where the emphasis is no longer on equilibrium but on the intrinsic dynamics of urban change. Even these views, however, imply a conventional wisdom where the real focus of urban studies is on processes that lead to comparatively slow changes in urban organization, where the functions determining such change are very largely routine, accomplished over months or years, rather than any lesser cycle of time. There is a tacit assumption that longer term change subsumes routine change on a day-to-day or hour-by-hour basis, which is seen as simply supporting the fixed spatial infrastructures that we perceive cities to be built around. Transportation modeling, for example, is fashioned from this standpoint in that routine trip-making behavior is the focus of study, its explanation being central to the notion that spatial structures are inert and long lasting.

76. We, according to the passage, tend to observe cities _____.
    A. chronologically
    C. sporadically
    B. longitudinally
    D. horizontally

77. We think about a city as _____.
    A. a spatial event
    C. a social environment
    B. a symbolical world
    D. an interrelated system

78. Cross-sectional studies show that cities _____.
    A. are structured in three dimensions
    B. are transformed rapidly in any aspect
    C. are resilient and long lasting through time
    D. change slowly in spatial and social structures

79. The author is drawing our attention to _____.
    A. the equilibrium of urban spatial structures
    B. the intrinsic dynamics of urban change
    C. the fixed spatial infrastructure
    D. all of the above

80. The conventional notion, the author contends, _____.
    A. presents the inherent nature of a city
    B. underlies the fixed spatial infrastructures
    C. places an emphasis on lesser cycles of time
    D. hinders the physical change of urban structure

Passage Five

When it is sunny in June, my father gets in his first cutting of hay. He starts on the creek meadows, which are flat, sandy, and hot. They are his driest land. This year, vacationing from my medical practice, I returned to Vermont to help him with the haying.

The heft of a bale（大捆）through my leather gloves is familiar: the tautness of the twine, the heave of the bale, the sweat rivers that run through the hay chaff on my arms. This work has the smell of sweet grass and breeze. I walk behind the chug and clack of the baler, moving the bales into piles so my brother can do the real work of picking them up later. As hot as the air is, my face is hotter. I am surprised at how soon I get tired. I take a break and sit in the shade, watching my father bale, trying not to think about how old he is, how the heat affects his heart, what might happen.

This is not my usual work, of course. My usual work is to sit with patients and listen to them. Occasionally I touch them, and am glad that my hands are soft. I don't think my patients would like farmer callous and dirty hands on their tender spots. Reluctantly I feel for lumps in breasts and testicles, hidden swellings of organs and joints, and probe all the painful places in my patients' lives. There are many. Perhaps I am too soft, could stand callous of a different sort.

I feel heavy after a day's work, as if all my patients were inside me, letting me carry them. I don't mean to. But where do I put their stories? The childhood beatings, ulcers from stress, incapacitating depression, fears, illness? These are not my experiences, yet I feel them and carry them with me. I search out these stories in my patients, try to recognize them, try to find healthier meanings. I spent the week before vacation crying.

The hay field is getting organized. Piles of three and four bales are scattered around the field. They will be easy to pick up. Dad climbs, tired and lame, from the tractor. I hand him a jar of ice water, and he looks with satisfaction on his job just done. I'll stack a few more bales and maybe drive the truck for my brother. My father will have some appreciative customers this winter, as he sells his bales of hay.

I've needed to feel this heaviness in my muscles, the heat on my face. I am taunted by the simplicity of this work, the purpose and results, the definite boundaries of the fields, the dimensions of the bales, for illness is not defined by the boundaries of bodies; it spills into families, homes, schools, and my office, like hay tumbling over the edge of the cutter bar. I feel the rough stubble left in its wake. I need to remember the stories I've helped reshape, new meanings stacked against the despair of pain. I need to remember the smell of hay in June.

81. Which of the following is NOT true according to the story?

   A. The muscular work in the field has an emotional impact on the narrator.

   B. The narrator gets tired easily working in the field.

   C. It is the first time for the narrator to do haying.

   D. The narrator is as physician.

82. In retrospection, the narrator _____.

   A. feels guilty before his father and brother

   B. defends his soft hands in a meaningful way

   C. hates losing his muscular power before he knows it

   D. is shamed for the farmer callous he does not possess

83. As a physician, the narrator is _____.

   A. empathic   B. arrogant

   C. callous   D. fragile

84. His associations punctuate _____.

   A. the similarities between medicine and agriculture

   B. the simplicity of muscular work

   C. the hardship of life everywhere

   D. the nature of medical practice

85. The narrator would say that _____.

   A. it can do physicians good to spend a vacation doing muscular work

   B. everything is interlinked and anything can be anything

   C. he is a shame to his father

   D. his trip is worth it

Passage Six

Everyone has seen it happen. A colleague who has been excited, involved, and productive slowly begins to pull back, lose energy and interest, and becomes a shadow or his or her former self. Or, a person who has been a beacon of vision and idealism retreats into despair or cynicism. What happened? How does someone who is capable and committed become a person who functions minimally and does not seem to care for the job or the people that work there?

Burnout is a chronic state of depleted energy, lack of commitment and involvement, and continual frustration, often accompanied at work by physical symptoms, disability claims and performance problem. Job burnout is a crisis of spirit, when work that was once exciting and meaningful becomes deadening. An organization's most valuable resource—the energy, dedication, and creativity of its employees—is often squandered by a climate that limits or frustrates the pool of talent and energy available.

Milder forms of burnout are a problem at every level in every type of work. The burned-out manager comes to work, but he brings a shell rather than a person. He experiences little satisfaction, and feels uninvolved, detached, and uncommitted to his work and co-workers. While he may be effective by external standards, he works far below his own level of productivity. The people around him are deeply affected by his attitude and energy level, and the whole community begins to suffer.

Burnout is a crisis of the spirit because people who burn out were once on fire. It's especially scary and consequential because it strikes some of the most talented. If they can't maintain their fire, others ask, who can? Are these people lost forever, or can the inner flame be rekindled? People often feel that burnout just comes upon them and that they are helpless victims of it. Actually, the evidence is growing that there were ways for individuals to safeguard and renew their spirit, and, more important, there are ways for organizations to change conditions that lead to burnout.

86. The passage begins with _____.
    A. a personal transition
    B. a contrast between two types of people
    C. a shift from conformity to individuality
    D. a mysterious physical and mental state

87. Which of the following is related with the crisis of spirit?
    A. Emotional exhaustion.
    B. Depersonalization.
    C. Reduced personal accomplishment.
    D. All of the above.

88. Job burnout is a crisis of spirit, which will result in _____.
    A. a personal problem
    B. diminished productivity
    C. an economic crisis in a country
    D. a failure to establish a pool of talent and energy

89. Burnout can be _____.
    A. fatal
    B. static
    C. infectious
    D. permanent

90. Those who are burned-out, according to the passage, are potentially able _____.
    A. to find a quick fix
    B. to restore what they have lost
    C. to be aware of their status quo
    D. to challenge their organization

GO TO THE NEXT PAGE FOR PAPER TWO: WRITING.

PAPER TWO

Part Ⅴ　Writing (20%)

Directions: *In this part, there is a passage in Chinese. Read it carefully and then translate it into English. Please write your answer on the* **ANSWER SHEET**.

答题要求

（1）忠实原文，不能随意发挥；

（2）用词恰当，注意词性的必要转换；

（3）英语语法使用恰当；

（4）文字通顺、符合英语表达习惯。

　　政府有关专家指出，奥密克戎绝不等同于大号流感，中国具备实现"动态清零"的能力和条件，坚持"动态清零"总方针不动摇，最大限度保障了人民生命安全和经济社会发展。

　　他还指出，衡量一个病毒的严重程度要综合考虑传播力和所导致的重症和死亡，奥密克戎的传播力远大于流感和此前的新冠其他变异株。在没有防护措施的情况下，平均一个人可以传播 9.5 个人。从病死率来看，全球的流感平均病死率为 0.1%，而奥密克戎变异株在真实世界的数据显示其平均病死率是 0.75%，约为流感的 7～8 倍，老年人群病死率超过 10%，是普通流感的近百倍。"动态清零"的核心是在当前无法消灭病毒也无法彻底阻止感染发生的情况下，对疫情发现一起扑灭一起。

THIS IS THE END OF THIS OFFICIAL TEST.

Hi-Fi FATMD Test 2
Answer Keys
（非标准答案，仅供参考）

Part Ⅰ. Listening

1-3: BCA   4-6: DAC   7-9: ADC   10-12: CBA   13-15: CAB   16-18: ACB   19-21: ADD

22-24: CCD   25-27: DBC   28-30: BBA

Part Ⅱ. Vocabulary

31-35: CABAA   36-40: CCDAD   41-45: BACBA   46-50:ABDCB

Part Ⅲ. Cloze

51-55: BDABD   56-60: BBBCB

Part Ⅳ. Reading

61-65: BCBBC   66-70: BDABC   71-75: CACDB   76-80: BADDA   81-85: ACBAA

86-90:DCBCB

Part Ⅴ. Translation Sample

A government health expert pointed out that Omicron is in noway comparable to a major influenza. China, having the ability and resources to achieve "dynamic zero-case", will unswervingly adhere to this policy to ensure the safety of people's lives and economic and social developments to the greatest extent.

He also pointed out that to measure the severity of a virus, we should comprehensively consider its transmission power, severity and death rate it might cause. Omicron's transmission power is much greater than that of influenza and other variants of the previous COVID-19. Without protective measures, an average person can transmit the virus to an average of 9.5 persons. In terms of morbidity and mortality, the global average morbidity and mortality rate for influenza is 0.1%, while the real-world data for the Omicron variant shows that its average morbidity and mortality rate is about 0.75%, which is about 7 to 8 times higher than that of influenza, and the morbidity and mortality rate for the elderly population is over 10%, which is nearly 100 times higher than that of an ordinary influenza. The core of "the dynamic zero-case policy" is to eliminate the virus and prevent the virus from spreading. (192 words)

Tapescript for the Listening Comprehension

Section A

Conversation One (Word Count: 98)

DR: Right, then. Let's finish the rest of the examination, and then we'll check the pressure again. Would you sit up a bit more for me, so I can listen to your heart. (1. A) That's fine. Breathe in ... breathe out ... hold it ... breathe away. Now would you turn on your left side, please? Good. Lie right out ... okay. Sit up again, please. Lean forward. Breathe away quietly through your mouth. Say ninety-nine.(2. B)

MR Jenkins: Ninety-nine.

DR: A couple of times more.(2. B)

MR Jenkins: Ninety-nine, ninety-nine, ninety-nine–

DR: Good. Just one or two other things, then, and we'll have a look at that blood pressure again.(3. C)

Questions 1 to 3 are based on the conversation you have just heard.

1. What are the two speakers doing?   A)（主旨概括）
2. What does the doctor ask the patient to say repeatedly?   B)（具体细节）
3. What will the doctor probably do after this conversation? C)（判断推理）

Conversation Two (Word Count: 127)

M: History Department, Dr. Bezel speaking.

W: Hello, Professor Bezel. This is Janie Bob calling. My roommate, Jim McLean, is a graduate assistant in your department. Jim asked me to call you because he has a throat infection (4. D) and he can't talk to you himself. (5. A)

M: A throat infection? That's a pity. Is there something I can do to help?

W: In fact, he has class this afternoon from one-thirty to three, and he won't make it. He doesn't want to cancel the class completely though.

M: Is he looking for a substitute?

W: No, that actually wouldn't be necessary. What he wants me to do is find someone to go in and play a ninety-minute wildlife videotape about native North American rodents. (6. C) It should only take a few minutes to set up.

Questions 4~6 are based on the conversation you've just heard.

4. What is Jim's problem?   D)（具体细节）
5. Why can't Jim come to give the class?   A)（具体细节）
6. What does Jim want someone to do for him?   C)（具体细节）

Conversation Three (Word Count: 131)

M: Oh, it's you, Miss Bramley. Come in and sit down. Now, what was it? Oh, yes, your ankle. Has there been any improvement since last week? (7. A)

W: Well, no. I'm afraid not, doctor. The leg's still the same.

M: I'd better have another look at it. Hm. It's still very swollen. (8. D) Have you been resting it, as I told you to?

W: It's so difficult to rest it, doctor, you know, with a house to run, and six children and...

M: Well, I've given you my advice. I'm sorry, but rest is necessary; otherwise, I wouldn't have insisted on it. You must sit for at least four hours a day with the leg raised; otherwise, the ankle isn't going to improve. (9. C) You understand that?

W: Yes, I understand, and I'll try to do as you say.

Questions 7~9 are based on the conversation you've just heard.

7. When did the woman see the man last time?   A)（判断推理）
8. What's wrong with the woman?   D)（具体细节）
9. What advice did the man give the woman?   C)（具体细节）

Conversation Four (Word Count: 166)

M: How's your toothache? (10. C)

W: It's gone, thanks. I went to the dentist last night and he took care of it.

M: Which tooth was it?

W: The last one on the upper right-hand side. It has a huge filling in it now.

M: I hate having my teeth filled. It's not just the pain I hate. It's the sound of drilling.

W: So do I. I'd rather have a tooth pulled than filled.

M: Have you ever had one of your teeth pulled?

W: No, but the one the dentist just filled will have to come out someday. He says it can't be filled again. (11. B)

M: Teeth keep causing trouble, and nobody really does anything about it. (12. A) I can't understand why.

W: They can put men on the moon, but they can't keep people from having trouble with their teeth.

M: They can give somebody a different heart. Why can't they give him different teeth?

W: I've heard they're working on that.

M: On second thought, I'm not sure I'd want to eat with some other person's teeth.

Questions 10~12 are based on the conversation you've just heard.

10. What is the dialogue mainly about?   C)（主旨概括）

11. Which of the following statements is true according to the conversation?   B)（具体细节）

12. What does the man complain of?   A)（判断推理）

Conversation Five (Word Count: 160)

W: You'll never believe what I heard on "EcoWatch" last night.

M: Try me.

W: Supposedly some researchers have found evidence for communication among trees. (13. C)

M: Please. You must be kidding.

W: I swear it's what they said. Apparently, those ecologists were studying a group of willow trees that were infested with caterpillars. They were in the process of trying to cure the trees when...

M: When the trees started talking to them?

W: No, listen. One particular tree cured itself. It managed to change the chemistry of its leaves so that the caterpillars couldn't stand the taste.

M: Hmm, I'm impressed that the trees know how to take care of themselves, but that doesn't really mean they... (14. A)

W: If you'd let me finish then you'd understand. After the first tree had successfully altered the chemistry of its leaves, it produced a strange smell (15. B); shortly thereafter the surrounding trees which had not yet become infected began to undergo similar metamorphoses(变形)---their leaves also began to produce this strange smell.

Questions 13~15 are based on the conversation you've just heard.

13. What was the focus of the TV program the woman saw?   C)（主旨概括）

14. What is the man's attitude towards the woman's remarks about research finding?   A)（判断推理）

15. According to the conversation, what happened to the willow trees first?   B)（具体细节）

Section B

Passage One (Word Count: 110)

Reducing the amount of sleep students get at night has a direct impact on their performance at school during the day.(16. A) According to classroom teachers, elementary and middle school students who stay up late exhibit more learning and attention problems. This has been shown by a Brown Medical School and Bradley Hospital research. In the study, teachers were not told the amount of sleep students received when completing weekly performance reports, yet they rated the students who had received eight hours or less as having the most trouble recalling all the material, learning new lessons and completing high-quality work. (17. C) Teachers also reported that these students had more difficulty paying attention. (18. B)

Questions 16~18 are based on the passage you've just heard.

16. What is the passage mainly about?   A)（主旨概括）

17. What were teachers told to do in the experiment?   C)（判断推理）

18. According to the experiment, what problem can insufficient sleep cause in students?   B)（具体细节）

Passage Two (Word Count: 150)

Katherine Stothard and colleagues from Britain's Newcastle University combined data from 18 studies to look at the risk of abnormalities of babies whose mothers were obese or overweight. (19. A; 20. D) The study found obese women were nearly twice as likely to have a baby with neural tube defects, which caused by the incomplete development of the brain or spinal cord. For one such defect, spina bifida(脊柱裂), the risk more than doubled. The researchers also detected increased chances of heart defect, cleft lip, and palate, water on the brain and problems in the growth of arms and legs.

The World Health Organization classifies around 400 million people around the world as obese (21. D), including 20 million under the age of five, and the number is growing. Obesity raises the risks of diseases such as type 2 diabetes, heart problems and is a health concern piling pressure on already overburdened national health system.

Questions 19~21 are based on the passage you've just heard.

19. What is the main topic of the passage?　　　　　　　　　　　　　　　A)（主旨概括）
20. What can we learn about the birth defects in the talk?　　　　　　　　　D)（判断推理）
21. According to WHO, how many people are classified as obese around the world?　　D)（具体细节）

Passage Three (Word Count: 113)

In today's class, we'll be looking into some of the earliest publications of the Merck pharmaceutical corporation. (24. D) These late-nineteenth century pharmaceutical texts were some of the first used in the American West. Since there texts predate the United States Pharmacopeia handbooks, I think it is fair to say that these books served as the basis for drugs which were administered to hundreds of thousands of Americans during the late 1800's. (22. C)

It was because the medical facilities were frequently so lacking that these books were particularly essential. I'd like you to take note of the simplicity of the language used to describe the procedures and the emphasis on practical issues in the lab notes. (23. C)

Questions 22~24 are based on the passage you've just heard.

22. What are the pharmaceutical books the professor is displaying?　　　　　C)（判断推理）
23. What does the professor ask the students to pay attention to in the books?　　C)（具体细节）
24. Which of the following pharmaceutical corporations published these books?　　D)（具体细节）

Passage Four (Word Count: 206)

For today's lab quiz (26. B) I have brought a flask of liquid nitrogen to class so I would like you to be particularly careful if you are near the front desk. (25. D) I'll show you why you need to be careful in the next few minutes. But first, let's discuss some of the properties of this material.

The liquid in this apparently smoking canister is cooled to below 210 degrees Celsius because at a higher temperature Nitrogen is a gas. The vapors that rise from the canister are harmless as they consist of water vapour and evaporating nitrogen which is non-toxic; in fact, as you know very well, nitrogen is the most common element in the atmosphere, occupying approximately 70% of the air we breathe.

Indeed, this noble gas is among the most unreactive in its common gaseous state, but in its liquid state which is artificially created by means of powerful compressors it can produce some amazing results. Take this pencil for instance, when I pull it out the flask with these tongs, it seems normal enough, but as I drop it on the desk—it shatters. This effect is made possible by the extreme cold within the canister which freezes the pencil into a brittle state. (27. C)

Questions 25~27 are based on the passage you've just heard.

25. What is the main topic of this lecture?　　　　　　　　　　　　　　D)（主旨概括）

26. Why did the professor bring the liquid nitrogen to class?　　　　　　B)（具体细节）

27. Why did the pencil shatter when it dropped?　　　　　　　　　　　C)（判断推理）

Passage Five (Word Count: 165)

Americans are suffering from a serious sleep deficit while also cutting back on leisure activities as they spend more time at work. (28. B) A world that "never goes to sleep" offers many diverse activities, but encourages unhealthy and sometimes anti-social lifestyles for America's adults. Instead of working to live, they are living to work, a shift that has had a profound impact on their personal lives. Adults report spending less time sleeping, whilst engaging in more social and leisure activities. Most Americans say they suffer from sleep problems and when they go to sleep, many sleep alone even if they are married. These are some of the key findings in the National Sleep Foundation's 2001 "Sleep in America" poll, which looks at the relationship between Americans' lifestyles, sleep habits and sleep problems. Sleep deprivation continues to be widespread in America. According to the NSF poll, 63% of American adults do not get the recommended eight hours of sleep needed for good health, safety, and optimum performance. (29. B) (30. A)

Questions 28~30 are based on the passage you've just heard.

28. What does the host attribute sleep deprivation to?　　　　　　　　B)（主旨概括）

29. What proportion of Americans does not get enough sleep?　　　　　　B)（具体细节）

30. How many hours of sleep are recommended for good health?　　　　　A)（具体细节）

Hi-Fi FATMD Test 3

国家医学考试中心标准答题卡

姓　名	
准考证号	
报考学校	

考生须知

1.答题前，考生务必用黑色字迹签字笔或水笔将姓名、准考证号、报考学校填写清楚。
2.按照题号顺序在各题目的答题区域内作答，未在对应的答题区域作答或超出答题区域的作答均不给分。
3.选择题用2B铅笔作答，不得使用涂改液。

条形码粘贴框

填涂说明　正确填涂 ●　错误填涂 ⊘⊗◎◍⊖

缺考违纪标记栏：　缺考 ○　作弊 ○　（此项由监考人员填涂！）

选择题

1	Ⓐ Ⓑ Ⓒ Ⓓ Ⓔ	16	Ⓐ Ⓑ Ⓒ Ⓓ Ⓔ	31	Ⓐ Ⓑ Ⓒ Ⓓ Ⓔ	46	Ⓐ Ⓑ Ⓒ Ⓓ Ⓔ	61	Ⓐ Ⓑ Ⓒ Ⓓ Ⓔ	76	Ⓐ Ⓑ Ⓒ Ⓓ Ⓔ
2	Ⓐ Ⓑ Ⓒ Ⓓ Ⓔ	17	Ⓐ Ⓑ Ⓒ Ⓓ Ⓔ	32	Ⓐ Ⓑ Ⓒ Ⓓ Ⓔ	47	Ⓐ Ⓑ Ⓒ Ⓓ Ⓔ	62	Ⓐ Ⓑ Ⓒ Ⓓ Ⓔ	77	Ⓐ Ⓑ Ⓒ Ⓓ Ⓔ
3	Ⓐ Ⓑ Ⓒ Ⓓ Ⓔ	18	Ⓐ Ⓑ Ⓒ Ⓓ Ⓔ	33	Ⓐ Ⓑ Ⓒ Ⓓ Ⓔ	48	Ⓐ Ⓑ Ⓒ Ⓓ Ⓔ	63	Ⓐ Ⓑ Ⓒ Ⓓ Ⓔ	78	Ⓐ Ⓑ Ⓒ Ⓓ Ⓔ
4	Ⓐ Ⓑ Ⓒ Ⓓ Ⓔ	19	Ⓐ Ⓑ Ⓒ Ⓓ Ⓔ	34	Ⓐ Ⓑ Ⓒ Ⓓ Ⓔ	49	Ⓐ Ⓑ Ⓒ Ⓓ Ⓔ	64	Ⓐ Ⓑ Ⓒ Ⓓ Ⓔ	79	Ⓐ Ⓑ Ⓒ Ⓓ Ⓔ
5	Ⓐ Ⓑ Ⓒ Ⓓ Ⓔ	20	Ⓐ Ⓑ Ⓒ Ⓓ Ⓔ	35	Ⓐ Ⓑ Ⓒ Ⓓ Ⓔ	50	Ⓐ Ⓑ Ⓒ Ⓓ Ⓔ	65	Ⓐ Ⓑ Ⓒ Ⓓ Ⓔ	80	Ⓐ Ⓑ Ⓒ Ⓓ Ⓔ
6	Ⓐ Ⓑ Ⓒ Ⓓ Ⓔ	21	Ⓐ Ⓑ Ⓒ Ⓓ Ⓔ	36	Ⓐ Ⓑ Ⓒ Ⓓ Ⓔ	51	Ⓐ Ⓑ Ⓒ Ⓓ Ⓔ	66	Ⓐ Ⓑ Ⓒ Ⓓ Ⓔ	81	Ⓐ Ⓑ Ⓒ Ⓓ Ⓔ
7	Ⓐ Ⓑ Ⓒ Ⓓ Ⓔ	22	Ⓐ Ⓑ Ⓒ Ⓓ Ⓔ	37	Ⓐ Ⓑ Ⓒ Ⓓ Ⓔ	52	Ⓐ Ⓑ Ⓒ Ⓓ Ⓔ	67	Ⓐ Ⓑ Ⓒ Ⓓ Ⓔ	82	Ⓐ Ⓑ Ⓒ Ⓓ Ⓔ
8	Ⓐ Ⓑ Ⓒ Ⓓ Ⓔ	23	Ⓐ Ⓑ Ⓒ Ⓓ Ⓔ	38	Ⓐ Ⓑ Ⓒ Ⓓ Ⓔ	53	Ⓐ Ⓑ Ⓒ Ⓓ Ⓔ	68	Ⓐ Ⓑ Ⓒ Ⓓ Ⓔ	83	Ⓐ Ⓑ Ⓒ Ⓓ Ⓔ
9	Ⓐ Ⓑ Ⓒ Ⓓ Ⓔ	24	Ⓐ Ⓑ Ⓒ Ⓓ Ⓔ	39	Ⓐ Ⓑ Ⓒ Ⓓ Ⓔ	54	Ⓐ Ⓑ Ⓒ Ⓓ Ⓔ	69	Ⓐ Ⓑ Ⓒ Ⓓ Ⓔ	84	Ⓐ Ⓑ Ⓒ Ⓓ Ⓔ
10	Ⓐ Ⓑ Ⓒ Ⓓ Ⓔ	25	Ⓐ Ⓑ Ⓒ Ⓓ Ⓔ	40	Ⓐ Ⓑ Ⓒ Ⓓ Ⓔ	55	Ⓐ Ⓑ Ⓒ Ⓓ Ⓔ	70	Ⓐ Ⓑ Ⓒ Ⓓ Ⓔ	85	Ⓐ Ⓑ Ⓒ Ⓓ Ⓔ
11	Ⓐ Ⓑ Ⓒ Ⓓ Ⓔ	26	Ⓐ Ⓑ Ⓒ Ⓓ Ⓔ	41	Ⓐ Ⓑ Ⓒ Ⓓ Ⓔ	56	Ⓐ Ⓑ Ⓒ Ⓓ Ⓔ	71	Ⓐ Ⓑ Ⓒ Ⓓ Ⓔ	86	Ⓐ Ⓑ Ⓒ Ⓓ Ⓔ
12	Ⓐ Ⓑ Ⓒ Ⓓ Ⓔ	27	Ⓐ Ⓑ Ⓒ Ⓓ Ⓔ	42	Ⓐ Ⓑ Ⓒ Ⓓ Ⓔ	57	Ⓐ Ⓑ Ⓒ Ⓓ Ⓔ	72	Ⓐ Ⓑ Ⓒ Ⓓ Ⓔ	87	Ⓐ Ⓑ Ⓒ Ⓓ Ⓔ
13	Ⓐ Ⓑ Ⓒ Ⓓ Ⓔ	28	Ⓐ Ⓑ Ⓒ Ⓓ Ⓔ	43	Ⓐ Ⓑ Ⓒ Ⓓ Ⓔ	58	Ⓐ Ⓑ Ⓒ Ⓓ Ⓔ	73	Ⓐ Ⓑ Ⓒ Ⓓ Ⓔ	88	Ⓐ Ⓑ Ⓒ Ⓓ Ⓔ
14	Ⓐ Ⓑ Ⓒ Ⓓ Ⓔ	29	Ⓐ Ⓑ Ⓒ Ⓓ Ⓔ	44	Ⓐ Ⓑ Ⓒ Ⓓ Ⓔ	59	Ⓐ Ⓑ Ⓒ Ⓓ Ⓔ	74	Ⓐ Ⓑ Ⓒ Ⓓ Ⓔ	89	Ⓐ Ⓑ Ⓒ Ⓓ Ⓔ
15	Ⓐ Ⓑ Ⓒ Ⓓ Ⓔ	30	Ⓐ Ⓑ Ⓒ Ⓓ Ⓔ	45	Ⓐ Ⓑ Ⓒ Ⓓ Ⓔ	60	Ⓐ Ⓑ Ⓒ Ⓓ Ⓔ	75	Ⓐ Ⓑ Ⓒ Ⓓ Ⓔ	90	Ⓐ Ⓑ Ⓒ Ⓓ Ⓔ

书面表达

请用黑色签字笔在答题区域内作答，超出黑色边框区域的答案无效！

样张（英语）

5

10

国家医学考试中心监制　　北京世纪互联软件开发有限公司设计制作　LT–1/8L 2019L146F

书 面 表 达　　　　　　　　请用黑色签字笔在答题区域内作答，超出黑色边框区域的答案无效！

15

20

25

30

LT-1/8R 2013B002B

Hi-Fi FATMD Test 3

PAPER ONE

Part I   Listening Comprehension (30%)

Section A

Directions: *In this section, you will hear fifteen short conversations between two speakers. At the end of each conversation, you will hear a question about what is said. The question will be read only once. After you hear the question, read the four possible answers marked A, B, C, and D. Choose the best answer and mark the letter of your choice on the* **ANSWER SHEET**.

Listen to the following example:

You will hear:

    W: I feel faint.

    M: No wonder. You haven't had a bite all day.

    Question: What's the matter with the woman?

You will read:

    A. She is sick.

    B. She was bitten by an ant.

    C. **She is hungry.**

    D. She spilled her paint.

    Here C is the right answer.

Sample Answer

A B ● D

Now let's begin with question Number 1.

1.   A. To do some experiments.   B. To attend a class.
    C. To review his lessons.   D. To take a test.

2.   A. In a hotel.   B. In the hospital.
    C. In the prison.   D. At the airport.

3.   A. He got an ulcer in his stomach.   B. He got hurt in the soccer game.
    C. He will be discharged soon.   D. He got his tumor removed.

4.   A. She told a lie so as not to hurt Jimmy.   B. She left because she had a headache.
    C. She hurt Jimmy by telling him a lie.   D. She slept off her headache.

5.   A. His new car is not fast enough.   B. His new car moves very fast.
    C. His new car is a real bargain.   D. His new car is somewhat of a financial burden.

6.   A. Get more time to relax.   B. Take some tranquilizers.
    C. Seek a second opinion.   D. Avoid her responsibilities.

7.   A. He got a headache while establishing the institute.
    B. He had a hard time getting the institute started.

C. Everything was OK at the beginning.

D. It is impossible to open such an institute in Seoul.

8. A. Excited.   B. Frustrated.

   C. Annoyed.   D. Relieved.

9. A. Each class lasts an hour.

   B. The class is meeting in an hour and a half.

   C. The class meets four hours and a half per week.

   D. The class meets for half an hour three times a week.

10. A. The woman was a good skier.   B. The woman couldn't ski.

    C. The woman didn't intend to go skiing.   D. The woman didn't like Swiss.

11. A. She's an insurance agent.   B. She's an insurance client.

    C. She's a bank clerk.   D. She's a driver.

12. A. He tripped over some crutches.   B. He had rheumatism in his legs.

    C. He sprained his foot.   D. He broke his leg.

13. A. The vacation is almost gone.   B. The vacation has just started.

    C. They are prepared for the new semester.   D. They can't wait for the new semester.

14. A. She was knocked down by a feather.   B. She was ashamed of Larry.

    C. She was really surprised.   D. She was proud of Larry.

15. A. To visit his son.   B. To perform an operation.

    C. To have an operation.   D. To send his son for an operation.

Section B

Directions: *In this section, you will hear one dialogue and two passages. After each one, you will hear five questions. After each question, read the four choices marked A, B, C, and D. Choose the best answer and mark the letter of your choice on the* **ANSWER SHEET**.

Sample Answer

A   B   ●   D

Dialogue

16. A. A pharmacist.   B. A visitor.

    C. A physician.   D. A dieter.

17. A. Cough.   B. Diarrhea.

    C. Headache.   D. Stomach upset.

18. A. Pain-killers.   B. Cough syrup.

    C. Antidiarrheals.   D. Indigestion tablets.

19. A. The cold weather.   B. Tiredness caused by traveling.

    C. The strange food he had eaten.   D. The greasy food he had eaten.

20. A. Take the medicine from the woman.   B. Go to see a specialist.

    C. Stop eating and drinking for a few days.   D. Stay in bed for a couple of days.

Passage One

21. A. Headaches.   B. Insomnia.

    C. Respiratory problems.   D. Digestive problems.

22. A. On Monday in Edinburgh.   B. On Wednesday in Edinburgh.

    C. On Monday at Staffordshire University.   D. On Wednesday at Staffordshire University.

23. A. 94.   B. 41.

C. 130.   D. 135.

24. A. The subjects were asked to write of their free will.

    B. The subjects were asked to write in a systematic way.

    C. The subjects were asked to say how often they made entries.

    D. The subjects were asked if they had written down anything traumatic.

25. A. The diarists who write of their free will.

    B. The diarists who were students at Staffordshire University.

    C. The diarists who had written about trauma.

    D. The non-diarists who were susceptible to headaches.

Passage Two

26. A. A brief history of British pubs.

    B. Beer-the British national drink.

    C. Various attempts made to curb drinking in Britain.

    D. The frustrating opening and closing hours of British pubs.

27. A. As early as 659 AD.   B. After 659 AD.

    C. Before the Roman invasion.   D. After the Roman invasion.

28. A. To restrict drinking hours.

    B. To restrict travelers to certain drinks.

    C. To encourage the locals to drink in other towns.

    D. To encourage inns to lodge various kinds of people.

29. A. People were better off.

    B. The government failed to persuade people from drinking.

    C. There appeared a new cheap drink.

    D. Drinkers had found various ways to get around the laws.

30. A. The licensing hours have been extended.

    B. Old people are not allowed to drink in pubs.

    C. Children are not allowed yet to drink in pubs.

    D. Big changes have taken place in pubs.

Part II   Vocabulary (10%)

Section A

Directions: *In this section all the sentences are incomplete. Beneath each of them are given four words or phrases, marked A, B, C, and D. Choose the word or phrase that best completes the sentence. Then, mark the letter of your choice on the* **ANSWER SHEET***.*

31. The doctor gave him an injection in order to _____ the pain.

    A. alleviate   B. aggregate

    C. abolish   D. allocate

32. His broken arm healed well, but she died of the pneumonia which followed as a _____.

    A. complement   B. compliment

    C. complexion   D. complication

33. Unfortunately, our vacation plans _____ on account of transport strike.

    A. fell back   B. fell through

    C. fell upon   D. fell to

34. The _____ climate of Hawaii attracts visitors from all over the world every year.
    A. genial   B. frigid
    C. genuine   D. foul

35. This is the _____ in which the organism lives most effectively.
    A. optimum   B. option
    C. ordeal   D. orbit

36. The doctor suggests that a good holiday in the country should _____ him _____ nicely after his operation.
    A. set...out   B. set...up
    C. set...off   D. set...aside

37. His behavior was so _____ that even the merciful people could not forgive him.
    A. unique   B. unconventional
    C. brutal   D. brilliant

38. _____ to your present job until you can get a better one.
    A. Hang about   B. Hang back
    C. Hang behind   D. Hang on

39. Suffering from his leg illness, Tom is very _____ nowadays.
    A. emaciated   B. eligible
    C. elastic   D. exceptional

40. He saved some money for artistic _____ such as fine paintings.
    A. donations   B. profits
    C. luxuries   D. lures

Section B

Directions: *Each of the following sentences has a word or phrase underlined. Beneath each sentence there are four words or phrases marked A, B, C, and D. Choose the word or phrase which can best keep the meaning of the original sentence if it is substituted for the underlined part. Mark the letter of your choice on the* **ANSWER SHEET**.

41. It has been proved that the chemical is lethal to rats but safe for cattle.
    A. fatal   B. reactive
    C. unique   D. vital

42. To their surprise, she has been nominated as candidate for the presidency.
    A. recognized   B. defined
    C. appointed   D. promoted

43. We cannot look down upon our opponent, who is an experienced swimmer.
    A. player   B. competitor
    C. referee   D. partner

44. She is regarded as a good nurse in that she attends to patients without any complaint.
    A. sees through   B. looks over
    C. takes in   D. cares for

45. It is well known that the minimum penalty for this crime is 2 years' imprisonment.
    A. conviction   B. span
    C. mercy   D. punishment

46. The whole area of the national and local governments tried to wipe out rats to prevent the spread of disease.

A. exterminate
B. dominate
C. determinate
D. contaminate

47. All the students are afraid of him since he is always <u>severe</u> with them.
    A. vigorous
    B. rigorous
    C. vigilant
    D. rigid

48. The biggest engineering project that they undertook was <u>encumbered</u> by lack of funds.
    A. cancelled
    B. condensed
    C. hampered
    D. haunted

49. In order to be a successful diplomat you must be enthusiastic and <u>magnetic</u>.
    A. arrogant
    B. industrious
    C. zealous
    D. attractive

50. He is successful as a doctor because of his <u>dynamic</u> personality, he seems to have unlimited energy.
    A. meticulous
    B. vigorous
    C. aggressive
    D. arbitrary

Part Ⅲ   Cloze (10%)

Directions: *In this section there is a passage with ten numbered blanks. For each blank, there are four choices marked A, B, C, and D on the right side. Choose the best answer and mark the letter of your choice on the* **ANSWER SHEET**.

Many Canadians enjoy the luxury of a large amount of living space. Canada is vast, and the homes are large according to the standards of many countries. Even __51__ inner cities do not reach the extremes found in other parts of world.

51. A. spacious   B. crowded
    C. remote   D. deserted

Canadians appreciate the space and value their privacy. Since families are generally small, many Canadian children enjoy the luxury of their own bedroom. Having more than one bathroom in a house is also considered a modern __52__.

52. A. convenience   B. comfort
    C. architecture   D. taste

Many rooms in Canadian homes have specialized functions. "Family rooms" are popular features in modern houses; these are __53__ "living rooms" since many living rooms have become reserved for entertaining. Some homes have formal and informal dining areas, __54__.

53. A. in common   B. in particular
    C. in chief   D. in fact

54. A. either   B. as well
    C. in turn   D. instead

Recreational homes are also popular __55__ Canadians. Some Canadians own summer homes, cottages, or camps. These may __56__ from a small one-room cabin to a luxurious building that rivals the comforts of the regular residence. Some cottages are winterized for year-round use. Cottages offer people the chance to "get away from it all." They are so popular that summer weekend traffic jams are

55. A. to   B. in
    C. with D. for

56. A. transform   B. convert
    C. range   D. shift

common, especially in large cities such as Toronto, where the number of people leaving town on Friday night and returning Sunday night ___57___ the highways for hours.

57. A. blocks   B. halts
     C. cuts off   D. keeps off

Sometimes, living in Canada means not only having privacy, but also being isolated. Mobility has become a part of modern life; people often do not live in one place long enough to ___58___ to know their neighbors. Tenants live their own lives in their apartments or townhouses. Even in private residential areas, where there is some ___59___, neighborhood life is not as close-knit as it once was. There seems to be ___60___ of a communal spirit. Life today is so hectic that there is often little time.

58. A. become   B. come
     C. get   D. grow

59. A. stability   B. mobility
     C. reality   D. tranquility

60. A. bit   B. much
     C. more   D. less

Part IV Reading Comprehension (30%)

Directions: *In this part there are six passages, each of which is followed by five questions. For each question there are four possible answers marked A, B, C, and D. Choose the best answer and mark the letter of your choice on the* **ANSWER SHEET**.

Passage One

The popular idea that classical music can improve your maths is falling from favor. New experiments have failed to support the widely publicized finding that Mozart's music promotes mathematical thinking.

Researchers reported six years ago that listening to Mozart brings about short-term improvements in spatial-temporal reasoning, the type of thinking used in maths. Gordon Shaw of the University of California at Irvine and Frances Rauscher of the University of Wisconsin in Oshkosh had asked students to perform spatial tasks such as imagining how a piece of paper would look if it were folded and cut in a certain pattern.

Some of the students then listened to a Mozart sonata and took the test again. The performance of the Mozart group got improved, Shaw found. He reasoned that listening to Mozart increases the number of connections between neurons.

But Kenneth Steele of Appalachian State University in North Carolina learnt that other studies failed to find this effect. He decided to repeat one of Shaw's experiments to see for himself.

Steele divided 125 students into three groups and tested their abilities to work out how paper would look if cut and folded. One group listened to Mozart, another listened to a piece by Philip Glass and the third did not listen to anything. Then the students took the test again.

No group showed any statistically significant improvement in their abilities. Steele concludes that the Mozart effect doesn't exist. "It's about as unproven and as unsupported as you can get," he says.

Shaw, however, defends his study. One reason he gives is that people who perform poorly in the initial test get the greatest boost from Mozart, but Steele didn't separate his students into groups based on ability. "We're still at the stage where it needs to be examined," Shaw says. "I suspect that the more we understand the neurobiology, the more we'll be able to design tests that give a robust effect."

61. It has been recently found out that _____.

   A. Mozart had an aptitude of music because of his mathematical thinking

    B. classical music cannot be expected to improve one's math

    C. the effects of music on health are widely recognized

    D. music favors one's mathematical thinking

62. Which of the following pairs, according to the widely publicized finding, is connected?

    A. Paper cutting and spatial thinking.

    B. The nature of a task and the type of thinking.

    C. Classical music and mathematical performance.

    D. Mathematical thinking and spatial-temporal reasoning.

63. In Shaw's test, the students would most probably _____.

    A. draw the image of the cut paper

    B. improve their mathematical thinking

    C. have the idea about classical music confirmed

    D. increase the number of neurons in their brains

64. From Steele's experiment we can say that _____.

    A. his hypothesis did not get proven and supported

    B. it was much more complicated than Shaw's

    C. the results were statistically significant

    D. Shaw's results were not repeatable

65. Shaw is critical of _____.

    A. Steele's results presented at a wrong Stage

    B. Steele's wrong selection of the testees

    C. Steele's ignorance of neurobiology

    D. Steele's test design

Passage Two

Long-suffering couples take heart. There is a good reason for those endless arguments in the front of the car: men and women use different parts of the brain when they try to find their way around, suggesting that the strategies they use might also be completely different.

Matthias Riepe and his colleagues at the University of Ulm in Germany asked 24 healthy volunteers— half of them men, half women—to find their way out of three virtual-reality mazes displayed on video goggles. Meanwhile, the researchers monitored the volunteers' brain activity using a functional magnetic resonance imaging (fMRI) scanner. This showed that men and women called on strikingly different brain areas to complete the task. "I didn't expect it to be so dramatic," says Riepe.

Previous studies have been shown that women rely mainly on landmarks to find their way. Men use these cues too, but they also use geometric cues, such as the angle and shape of a wall or a corner. Such studies also suggest that men navigate their way out of unfamiliar spaces more quickly, as Riepe found in his study, too.

Riepe discovered that both men and women used parts of the parietal cortex towards the top of the brain, the right side of the hippocampus and a few other well-established areas to find their way out. Neuroscientists think that the parietal regions help translate what the eyes see into information about where the body is in space, while the hippocampal region helps process how objects are arranged.

But other regions seemed to be exclusively male or female. The men engaged the left side of their hippocampus, which the researchers say could help with assessing geometry or remembering whether they have already visited a location. The women, by contrast, recruited their right frontal cortex.

Riepe says this may indicate that they were using their "working memory", trying to keep in mind the landmarks they had passed.

"It fits very well with the animal studies," says Riepe. He points out that there seem to be similar differences in rats. For example, damage to the frontal lobe will impair a female's sense of direction, but not a male's.

66. The studies on the driving issue have evolved _____.
    A. from the car to the driver
    B. from the reality to the virtual-reality
    C. from the physical cues to the parts of the brain
    D. from the cues of navigation to the strategies of driving

67. The different parts of the brain men and women use to find their way around, according to the passage, refer to _____.
    A. the left side of the hippocampus and the right frontal cortex
    B. the right and left side of their hippocampi respectively
    C. the right and left hemisphere of their brains respectively
    D. the parietal cortex and the hippocampus as a whole

68. The part of the brain women use may help explain why they _____.
    A. use geometric cues to navigate
    B. have a better memory than men
    C. rely mainly on landmarks to find their ways
    D. behave less aggressively than men in driving

69. The reason for the differences in the sexes, according to Riepe, could be _____.
    A. the environmental factor
    B. the psychological factor
    C. the innate factor
    D. all of the above

70. Which one of the following questions did the studies answer?
    A. How do women and men drive differently?
    B. How can we detect the brain activities during driving?
    C. Why do men and women argue over which route to take?
    D. Why does the damage to the frontal lobe impair the sense of direction?

Passage Three

Work has left you frazzled. Your legs ache when you get back from the gym...don't pop those aspirins just yet. Think hot springs. Cranking up a hot tub and hopping in is a natural remedy that can provide significant relief from physical pain and stress.

There are more than three million home spas in the U.S. today. There are numerous reasons spas have made the move from the decks of Hollywood producers to the back yards of middle America. Spas help reduce the effect of stress on your body, assist in muscle recovery, after the stress of exercise, and help heal muscles near arthritic joints.

There are three elements to hydrotherapy that, in tandem, provide these healing effects on the body: heat, buoyancy, and motion. When you exercise, your muscles develop thousands of microscopic tears which result in painful lactic acid build-up in the muscle tissue. Hydrotherapy's motion and warmth cause blood vessels to dilate, lowering blood pressure and speeding the flow of oxygen, endorphins, and cell-repairing nutrients to injured muscles. Additionally, buoyancy of the water reduces the strain on your knees and joints which allow the surrounding muscles to relax. This can be of crucial help to arthritis sufferers, because when joints are inflamed, the surrounding muscles become tense to protect them. Relaxing in a spa then makes your muscles more limber and reduces the pain. Water's healing potential has long been known.

We don't tend to associate intelligence with our bodies, yet as Thomas Edison said, "Great ideas originate in the muscles." Radical psychoanalyst Wilhelm Reich believed that many of us inhibit or deny impulses, feelings, traumas, and stresses by tightening our muscles and creating a kind of "body armor." He felt that as you cut off the source of pain, you also cut off the source of pleasure. By loosening body armor, by letting muscles relax, you can return to a feeling of flow and creativity.

Few things can relax the body more than a home spa. And a relaxed body leads to a relaxed mind. There is no better place to start relaxing than an hour in your home hot springs.

71. To begin with, what does the author insist we avoid doing?
    A. Undergoing physical pain and stress.　　B. Taking aspirin tablets.
    C. Going to the gym.　　D. Relaxing in a spa.

72. What does the second sentence in the second paragraph imply?
    A. The origin of spas.　　B. The popularity of hot springs.
    C. The flux of people to mid America.　　D. The spas as a luxury only for the rich.

73. After the stress of exercise, the injured muscles _____.
    A. will lead to arthritis
    B. contain plenty of microscopic tears
    C. can cause blood pressure to decline
    D. will boost the production of cell-repairing nutrients

74. The author contends that our creativity _____.
    A. can be enforced by the "body armor"
    B. does not occur in mind but in the muscles
    C. can be hampered with our muscles tightened
    D. is good only when we are free of mental and physical stress

75. Which of the following can be the best title for the passage?
    A. Spas, the Best Relaxation.　　B. A Brief History of Spas.
    C. Spa Resorts in the USA.　　D. Soak Away Stress.

Passage Four

Convincing the public to follow health advice can be tough and time-consuming. This may be why changes to health messages are often fiercely resisted by those whose job is to get the advice across. So, for example, the suggestion that smokers who cannot quit should reduce their exposure to harm by switching to chewing tobacco met with extreme opposition.

A still more ferocious debate is emerging over the health impact of sunshine. For the past 20 years, advice on sunlight has come from dermatologists who rightly warn people to cover up when they venture outside for fear of developing skin cancer. But evidence from researchers in other fields now suggests that short periods in the sun without protection—sometimes as little as a few minutes a day—can prevent most other major forms of cancer.

This surprising conclusion stems from findings that vitamin D, which is made by skin cells exposed to the sun's ultraviolet rays, is a potent anti-cancer agent. The researchers who made this discovery are eager to be heard. But their message is about as welcome as a bad rash, particularly in countries such as Australia and the US where fair-skinned immigrants living at Mediterranean latitudes have made skin cancer a huge

problem.

The American Academy of Dermatology argues that advocating one carcinogen—UV radiation—to protect against other forms of cancer is dangerous and misleading. If people need more vitamin D, they should take a multivitamin or drink milk fortified with it, says the academy. Unfortunately, the solution is not as simple as that. Critics also argue that the protective effect of sunlight is not yet proved. While this may be true, the evidence is very suggestive. The case is built on several studies that bring together cellular biology, biochemistry and epidemiology. And all the criticism of this theory counts for nothing if, as some of its advocates suggest, the number of people dying for lack of sunlight is four times as high as those dying from skin cancer. At the same time, those advocates must not overstate their case. Everyone wants to save as many lives as they can.

What we need now is for national medical research bodies and cancer research organizations to investigate the relative risks and benefits of sunshine. This will almost certainly mean more epidemiological work, which should start as soon as possible. As for the public: give them the facts, including risk estimates for short periods in the sun—and for covering up. It is patronizing（施恩于人的）to assume that people cannot deal with complex messages.

What we definitely do not want is a war of words between groups with polarized views, and no prospect of the issue being resolved. That way will only lead to confusion, distrust of doctors and more unnecessary deaths.

76. According to the first two paragraphs, the problem seems to be that the public _____.
    A. cannot be reached by health messages   B. is torn between two health messages
    C. never trust those health researchers   D. are divided over health problems

77. The recent opposition goes to _____.
    A. the protective value of sunshine
    B. the cancer-causing effect of sunshine
    C. the debate over the health impact of sunshine
    D. the two controversial messages about skin cancer

78. According to the critics, the health impact of sunshine _____.
    A. will be epidemiologically proved
    B. is misleading the public altogether
    C. merits a comprehensive investigation
    D. can be easily addressed with a simple solution

79. The author implies that health messages should be made easy _____.
    A. to debate   B. to swallow
    C. to estimate   D. to publicize

80. As for the issue, the author suggests that the public _____.
    A. decide on their own how much sunshine is too much
    B. avoid unnecessary deaths due to complex messages
    C. be provided with reliable and practicable messages
    D. facilitate the understanding of health messages

Passage Five

I make my way down the three chilly blocks to an old diner on Commercial Street. I am meeting a new friend for lunch. I've never been here before: this is not my part of town. And so I arrive early, to sit in an old wooden booth and learn what I can about the place.

They call it Katie's Kitchen. One hundred years ago, it was a bar. The barstools remain, but through community donations, it's now a respectable restaurant. The hostess, casher, and waiters are residents of a nearby hotel for the transient and unemployed and work here to gain dignity and job skills. Both the hotel and restaurant are run by Sister L, a nun with a heart and a great deal of business sense.

My new friend arrives. He works down the street, in a clinic for indigent（贫穷的）persons; he knows these people. The workers and many of the clients seem to know him too, for I see warmth and proud smiles on their faces as he greets them. Behind him, a few nameless souls wander in from the street in a swirl of December wind.

I focus on our waitress. A pretty girl of perhaps 18 years, she is all smiles and grace. I wonder for a moment why she's here—what her story is; what her dreams are; whether she is raising children on her own. But I cannot hold the thought, for she reminds me of another waitress at my favorite coffee shop—a college student with a bright future.

Some time later, I finish my soup and sandwich—a good meal made better because of the smile of the girl who served it. I wipe my mouth and go to pay. Eight dollars and sixty-four cents, for two. To our embarrassment, my friend and I discover that neither of us has cash, and my credit card is not good here. We sheepishly approach Sister L, who smiles and takes my bill. "It's okay," she says. "We'll buy your lunch. It'll be our pleasure."

Slowly, I leave the world of the diner. Back at the hospital where I work, my boss laments our financial woes. "We're really tight," he says. "The executive committee tells me we may not even have enough money to build the new critical care wing this year." He frowns, hesitates, then adds, "It's flu season, though, and perhaps by seeing patients in person rather than treating so many over the phone, we'll recoup some of our losses."

It's budget time, and I know that this means our gratis（免费的）fitness center memberships may be cancelled. We're in a tough bind.

Three streets away, a tattered man in a throwaway overcoat sits shivering in the diner. Sister L slowly fills his cup full of hot coffee. Holding the cup with trembling hands, he stares deeply into its dark center. There is healing in its rising steam.

81. The doctor in the story enters a restaurant which _____.
    A. has a one-hundred-year old bar   B. has won a reputation for its management
    C. performs charities among the immigrants   D. serves such respectable people as doctors

82. He happens to know that his new friend _____.
    A. has a great deal of business sense   B. is popular wherever he goes
    C. works as a clinical doctor   D. is a respectable person

83. What is it that he enjoys most at lunch?
    A. His associative memory.   B. The delicious soup and sandwich.
    C. The service by a beautiful waitress.   D. His sitting in an old wooden booth.

84. From the lunch bill to the hot coffee, we can see _____.
    A. Sister L's warm heart   B. financial woes everywhere
    C. the way the author looks at the world   D. indigent people's financial embarrassment

85. The doctor implies that they, as Sister L does, will _____.
    A. continue their healing despite their financial troubles
    B. expand their business despite tight budget
    C. avoid financial embarrassment
    D. treat more patients over the phone

Passage Six

Confronted with patient facing death, physicians may feel a sense of medical impotence and failure. Years of training and zeal to heal have focused on doing anything and everything to save the patient. Death is treated as the enemy. One might ask, "What use can I be if I cannot fix?" One may be tempted to withdraw. There may be no meaningful closure with a patient other than referral to home care or hospice.

Feelings evoked by a patient's dying are also antithetical（对立的）to the original "call" to medicine—the desire to make a difference in people's lives and the alleviation of pain and suffering. Over time these inner directives may have been obscured by the rigors of a pressured practice, not to mention the climate of malpractice litigation（诉讼）. This threat necessitates obsessive attention to the details of intervention options, possibly at the cost of considering the needs of the whole person at hand.

So the moment when death raises its specter（恐惧）is a crossroads. Herein lies the opportunity for physicians to go beyond their conventional model of relating to patients. This is when the conventional therapeutic tools can be set aside in favor of the most powerful contribution of all: the physician's caring itself. The only requirement is a willingness to extend conscious listening and basic humanity to the dying patient. The simple act of visitation, of presence, of taking the trouble to witness the patient's process can be in itself a potent healing affirmation—a sacramental（圣礼的）gesture received by the dying person who may be feeling helpless, diminished, and fearful that they have little to offer others. The patient may also fear that he or she has failed.

How meaningful it is to be told by my physicians that they are learning from me! I feel honored and joined by my physicians as we participate in these human, vulnerable, and mysterious moments at the end of my life. I and many dying persons would agree that beyond pain control, the three elements we most need are feeling cared about, being respected, and enjoining a sense of continuity, be it in relationships or in terms of spiritual awareness.

86. Facing a terminally-ill patient, physicians _____.
    A. have no right to withdraw
    B. must save him or her at any cost
    C. can do nothing but accept the failure
    D. can be caught in the dilemma of cure or care

87. During the pressured practice, the feelings evoked by a patient's dying _____.
    A. can lead to a legal suit
    B. are likely to be set aside
    C. tend to be antithetical to the quality of life
    D. urge the physician to save him or her by all means

88. According to the passage, the physician's caring relates to _____.
    A. the needs of the dying patient treated as a whole person
    B. the acceptance of medical impotence and failure
    C. the exploration of all the intervention options
    D. the avoidance of malpractice litigation

89. What the dying patient needs most that makes him or her feel honored is the physician's _____.
    A. willingness to perform the basic humane acts
    B. ability to alleviate pain effectively
    C. powerful healing competence
    D. frankness and honesty

90. Which of the following can be the best title for the passage?
    A. The Nature of Medicine.
    B. Medical Impotence and Failure.
    C. The Psychology of the Dying Patient.
    D. The Use of the Self as Medical Intervention.

GO TO THE NEXT PAGE FOR PAPER TWO: WRITING.

PAPER TWO

Part V Writing (20%)

Directions: *In this part there is an essay in Chinese. Read it carefully and then write a summary of 200 words in English on the **ANSWER SHEET**. Make sure that your summary covers all the major points of the article.*

答题要求

（1）紧扣主题，归纳总结；

（2）涵盖所有重要内容；

（3）避免选择原句进行简单翻译；

（4）无须推演或推论。

手术与害怕

外科疾病的治疗，多采用手术方法。而手术对于患者来说，是一次重大的不幸事件。因此手术本身就成为一种强烈的心理刺激，使患者处于焦虑、抑郁、紧张、恐惧等一系列情绪状态之中。情绪应激会引起一系列生理反应，促发与手术有关的心身症，如手术神经症、频发手术症、器官移植综合征等，以至严重影响手术的进行和手术的治疗效果。

手术包括治疗性手术，如创伤后的清创缝合、阑尾切除术、肾移植术、心脏冠状动脉旁路移植术等，以及诊断性手术，如剖腹探查、心导管检查、病理切片检查等，它们都是创伤性的治疗和检查方法。手术常常导致疼痛、大量出血及组织的损伤。这种刺激，常会使患者的生理和心理两方面都处于紧张状态，特别是有性格缺陷的患者，更易产生强烈的情绪反应，从而诱发心身症。如果医生能对其做一些解释和安慰，将会有效控制患者不良情绪的发展。

手术前患者强烈的情绪反应，可导致一系列的躯体反应，如心悸、气促、胸闷、出汗、失眠、血压升高、儿茶酚胺升高、交感神经兴奋等多种躯体反应。如果不做处理，势必影响手术的进行和效果，引起心身疾病或严重的精神障碍，还可诱发冠心病、脑血管疾病，造成手术意外。另外，由于情绪应激和手术创伤，引起促肾上腺皮质激素及皮质类固醇的分泌，会使免疫机制受到抑制，增加细菌感染的机会。

患者的情绪反应并不因手术的完成而中止，许多患者术后仍有强烈的情绪反应。术后的疼痛不适，身体活动不便，使患者情绪受到压抑，渴望他人给予情感上的关怀与支持。而医院单调的环境，手术后的恢复，以及对并发症的顾虑，可使患者情绪忧郁。此时家属、同事及医护人员的同情和怜悯，常使患者产生较强的依赖感。那些做过破坏性较强的手术，出现过严重并发症或被确诊为恶性肿瘤的患者常出现失望、抑郁的情绪。也有部分患者由于病痛被消除，常表现出愉快的情绪。

外科手术的情绪问题是可以预防及控制的。在手术前对患者进行心理情绪指导，学习情绪的自我调控方法，能有效地控制情绪对手术治疗的影响。许多患者都是首次做手术，由于对医院环境及手术过程不熟悉，以及不实际、不正确的想象，常使患者感到恐惧，此时可用脱敏疗法来帮助患者消除紧张，向患者讲解手术经过，也可播放一段类似手术的实况录像，让患者有一个直观的感受。对于那些公开暴露自己对手术恐惧，希望对手术有较多了解的患者，可让其反复观看同类录像，直到恐惧感缓解为止。对于病情较重，情绪反应强烈的患者可采用爱抚疗法。爱，有着异乎寻常的医疗效果，是消除情绪紧张、减轻思想负担的有效方法。美国洛杉矶医学院的专家们做了一次实验，他们对 54 位严重心律失常的男女患者进行观察，在每位手臂上安放一个心律测试仪，然后每天安排一位和蔼可亲的护士小姐 3

次到患者床前，握住他们的手，像是给他们拿脉，并温柔亲切地同患者交谈。实验结果显示，这些情绪不宁、充满死亡恐惧的患者，在女护士的爱抚体贴的几分钟内，心律竟出现平稳及安定，取得了药物治疗难以达到的效果。

　　人对于抚摸有着强烈的要求，婴儿被母亲抚摸能获得"安全感"，成人时期，爱人的爱抚和抚摸，能产生良好的生理及心理效应，达到消除不良情绪反应的作用。

THIS IS THE END OF THIS OFFICIAL TEST.

Hi-Fi FATMD Test 3
Answer Keys
（非标准答案，仅供参考）

Part Ⅰ. Listening

1-3: DBB   4-6: ADA   7-9: BDC   10-12: BAD   13-15: ACC   16-18: BAD   19-21: DAC

22-24: BDA   25-27: CAC   28-30: ACC

Part Ⅱ. Vocabulary

31-35: ADBAA   36-40: BCDAC   41-45: ACBDD   46-50: ADCDB

Part Ⅲ. Cloze

51-55: BADBC   56-60: CACAD

Part Ⅳ. Reading

61-65: BCBAB   66-70: CACCC   71-75: BBBDA   76-80: BBCDC   81-85: CDCAA

86-90: DDAAD

Part Ⅴ. Writing

Fears Caused by Surgical Operation

To most patients, surgical operation is never happy. As it causes fears and pains in most patients. This essay discusses fears caused by operation and how to deal with them.

Psychologically stimulating, operation makes patients worried, depressed, nervous and frightened. These emotional responses in turn cause physiological reactions such as operation necrosis, operation syndrome, and worst of all, they seriously affect the curative efficacy, process of the operation and the recovery. Fears before and after operation may cause many other bodily reactions, such as abnormal heartthrob, short breath, sweating, insomnia, hypertension, etc., which may in turn lead to physical and mental handicaps and accidents in operation.

To be sure, there are some ways to prevent fears and mental problems caused by operation. Doctors can give patients psychological advice, consultation and consolation. For example, some explanation and demonstration of operation may help patients relax and relieve. Gentle and tender caressing or stroking can also help patients calm down.

Conclusively, fears about operation may cause many problems and something done to it may help prevent the problems.

Tapescript for the Listening Comprehension

Section A

1. W: Where are you heading now? You seem to be in a bit of a hurry.

   M: I'm on my way to the biology building. I have an exam in about 20 minutes.

   W: What is the man going to do?   D)

2. M: Hello, I was wondering if Teller Smith has checked out yet.

   W: Just a moment. I will check with the Cancer Ward Desk.

   M: Thank you.

   W: Well, Mr. Smith is still here. But he will be released tomorrow.

　　M: Where is Mr. Smith now? B)

3. W: You know. Tom's been in a hospital for a couple of days.

　　M: And I am the one who put him there with my soccer moves.

　　W: Which of the following is true about Tom? B)

4. M: You left Jimmy's party early last night. Did you have a headache?

　　W: Well, I told Jimmy a white lie when I said I had to leave early because I had a headache.

　　M: What does the woman mean? A)

5. W: Your new car is fabulous.

　　M: Not so fast. I won't finish paying for it until 2010.

　　W: What does the man mean? D)

6. M: Well, I've checked you over pretty thoroughly and I can't find anything wrong. It sounds to me that you've been overdoing things.

　　W: Yes, I have.

　　M: I want you to take things easier. See if you can share your responsibilities so that you can make more time for yourself.

　　W: What does the man suggest the woman do? A)

7. W: I've heard that you've opened an institute of mental health in Seoul. How is it going?

　　M: Everything is ok now but it was quite a headache getting started.

　　W: What does the man mean? B)

8. M: Hi, Susan. How were your finals?

　　W: Hi, Dan. I finished my last exam this morning and my last term paper a few minutes ago. I really feel like I can see the light.

　　M: How was the woman feeling now? D)

9. W: Can you tell me how often the chemistry class meets?

　　M: It meets 3 times a week for an hour and a half each time.

　　W: What does the man mean? C)

10. M: You look freshened and energetic. Where did you go for the holiday?

　　W: I went to a skiing resort in Switzerland and had a wonderful time.

　　M: So, you can ski.

　　W: What had the man assumed? B)

11. W: Would you like to take car collision insurance?

　　M: No, thanks. I won't need any insurance.

　　W: What does the woman do? A)

12. W: Did you see Robert?

　　M: Yes, I did. His leg was in a cast and he was on crutches.

　　W: What happened to Robert? D)

13. W: I feel like it's only been a few days since the vacation started.

　　M: And it's almost time for the new semester.

　　W: What do the speakers mean? A)

14. M: Did you hear that Larry got a 630 on the TOEFL test?

　　W: You could have knocked me over with a feather.

　　M: What does the woman mean? C)

15. W: Good morning. Welcome to our ward. I'm Nurse Brown. Can I help you?

M: Yes, please. I'm Mr. Watson and this is my son Ricky who drove me here. I've come in for my operation.

W: Why did Mr. Watson come to the hospital?   C)

Section B
Dialogue

W: Good morning. Can I help you?

M: Yes, let's hope so. Thank God, you speak English.

W: Well, just a little. What seems to be wrong?

M: I've got an upset stomach. It's pretty bad. I've been up all night with it. Now, I've got a bad headache as well.

W: I see. When did it first start?

M: When I went to bed.

W: Do you think it's something you've eaten?

M: Oh, for sure. I'm not used to all this wining and dining.

W: Yes, you've really eaten a lot.

M: You can say that again.

W: Have you got diarrhea? Is it very loose?

M: That's what it feels like.

W: How often do you have to go?

M: I have to go every few minutes.

W: Are you drinking plenty of water? Bottled water?

M: I've had a few sips of water. I feel terribly thirsty.

W: Have you taken anything? Did you bring anything from home?

M: I've got only these indigestion tablets.

W: Can I see the packet?

M: Here you are. Look.

W: Have you taken anything for the headache?

M: I've taken a couple of paracetamol. That's all.

W: Do you feel tired?

M: Oh, now! I can hardly keep my eyes open.

W: Well, I think you've probably just eaten something a bit too rich for you. You know you are not used to it. I'm sure you will be all right in a couple of days with what I'm going to give you.

16. Which of the following best describes the man in the dialogue?   B)

17. The man suffered from the following symptoms EXCEPT _____.   A)

18. What medicine did the man bring with him from home?   D)

19. What might be the cause of the man's illness?   D)

20. What will the man probably do next?   A)

Passage One

Keeping a diary is bad for your health, say UK psychologists. They found that people who regularly keep a diary suffer from headaches, sleeplessness, digestive problems and social awkwardness more than people who don't. This finding challenges the assumption that people find it easier to get over a traumatic event if they write about it.

"We expected that diary keepers to have more benefits or be the same but they were worst off," says Elaine Duncan of Glasgow Caledonia University. "In fact, you will be probably much better off if you don't write anything at all." she adds.

The study carried out with David Sheffield of Staffordshire University was presented on Wednesday at a meeting of the British Psychological Society at Edinburgh. The peer studied 94 regular diarists, and compared their health with that of 41 non-diarists. The subjects, all students at Staffordshire University, answered questions about their diary keeping habits and filled in a standard questionaire. "We decided to test the idea that writing is cathartic," says Duncan. She claims that her study is the first to investigate subjects who write of their own free will.

In most other studies, volunteers are actually asked to write about traumatic experiences in a systematic way. The researchers asked the diarists recruited to say how often they made entries, and for how long they had kept diaries. They were also asked if they had written about anything traumatic. Statistically, the diarists scored much worse on health measures than the non-diarists. The worst affected of all were those who had written about trauma. "They were susceptible to headaches and the like." says Duncan.

21. According to UK psychologists, regular diarists are more likely to suffer from the following EXCEPT _____.   C)
22. When and where was Duncan study presented?   B)
23. How many subjects were there in Duncan study?   D)
24. What is special about Duncan study?   A)
25. According to Duncan study, who scored worst on health measures?   C)

Passage Two

Most foreigners find British pubs both fascinating and frustrating. Fascinating because they are unique to Great Britain and not at all like the bars you find in most other countries and frustrating because of their peculiar opening and closing hours. In fact, much of the long history of pub in Britain has to do with people who wanted to drink and others who wanted to stop them. The development of pubs and the laws surrounding them is an interesting way to learn a little more about our social history. Foreigners often think of tea as the British national drink. But compared to beer drinking, tea drinking is a very recent development. Beer has been drunk in Britain since before the Roman invasion. The earliest breweries were part of the monastery as early as 1659 AD, the king of Kent was making laws in an attempt to stop priests from getting drunk. By the late 16th century, drunkenness was a real problem and laws were passed to restrict drinking hours. In 1606 a law was passed which stated that the purpose of inns was to lodge wayfaring people only. Travelers were allowed to buy drinks at times forbidden to local people. However, the ingenuity of the dedicated drinkers got around this problem and the result was that the locals would simply move on to the next town or village when they wanted to continue drinking after time in their own village. In the 19th century, cheap gin appeared in Britain. It was very popular among poor people. Drunkenness again increased and more laws were passed. The temperate society was formed to fight against the deem in drink. This group of dedicated tea tried to persuade people to abstain from drinking by getting them to sign the pledge. In spite of various attempts to curb drinking or stamp it out completely, pubs continue to provide a major part of British social life. Their opening and closing hours are still restricted by laws although there have been recommendations recently for big changes. But nothing has happened yet, including extending licensing hours and admitting children.

26. What is this talk mainly about?   A)

27. When did people start to drink beer in Britain?   C)

28. What was the purpose of the law passed in 1606?   A)

29. Which of the following factors contributes to the rise of drunkenness in the 19th century?   C)

30. Which of the following is true about English pubs today?   C)

Hi-Fi FATMD Test 4

国家医学考试中心标准答题卡

姓　名	
准考证号	
报考学校	

考生须知

1.答题前，考生务必用黑色字迹签字笔或水笔将姓名、准考证号、报考学校填写清楚。

2.按照题号顺序在各题目的答题区域内作答，未在对应的答题区域作答或超出答题区域的作答均不给分。

3.选择题用2B铅笔作答，不得使用涂改液。

条形码粘贴框

填涂说明　　正确填涂 ●　　错误填涂 ⊘⊗⊙ ⊘⊙⊖

缺考违纪标记栏：　缺考 ○　　作弊 ○　　（此项由监考人员填涂！）

选择题

1 Ⓐ Ⓑ Ⓒ Ⓓ Ⓔ	16 Ⓐ Ⓑ Ⓒ Ⓓ Ⓔ	31 Ⓐ Ⓑ Ⓒ Ⓓ Ⓔ	46 Ⓐ Ⓑ Ⓒ Ⓓ Ⓔ	61 Ⓐ Ⓑ Ⓒ Ⓓ Ⓔ	76 Ⓐ Ⓑ Ⓒ Ⓓ Ⓔ
2 Ⓐ Ⓑ Ⓒ Ⓓ Ⓔ	17 Ⓐ Ⓑ Ⓒ Ⓓ Ⓔ	32 Ⓐ Ⓑ Ⓒ Ⓓ Ⓔ	47 Ⓐ Ⓑ Ⓒ Ⓓ Ⓔ	62 Ⓐ Ⓑ Ⓒ Ⓓ Ⓔ	77 Ⓐ Ⓑ Ⓒ Ⓓ Ⓔ
3 Ⓐ Ⓑ Ⓒ Ⓓ Ⓔ	18 Ⓐ Ⓑ Ⓒ Ⓓ Ⓔ	33 Ⓐ Ⓑ Ⓒ Ⓓ Ⓔ	48 Ⓐ Ⓑ Ⓒ Ⓓ Ⓔ	63 Ⓐ Ⓑ Ⓒ Ⓓ Ⓔ	78 Ⓐ Ⓑ Ⓒ Ⓓ Ⓔ
4 Ⓐ Ⓑ Ⓒ Ⓓ Ⓔ	19 Ⓐ Ⓑ Ⓒ Ⓓ Ⓔ	34 Ⓐ Ⓑ Ⓒ Ⓓ Ⓔ	49 Ⓐ Ⓑ Ⓒ Ⓓ Ⓔ	64 Ⓐ Ⓑ Ⓒ Ⓓ Ⓔ	79 Ⓐ Ⓑ Ⓒ Ⓓ Ⓔ
5 Ⓐ Ⓑ Ⓒ Ⓓ Ⓔ	20 Ⓐ Ⓑ Ⓒ Ⓓ Ⓔ	35 Ⓐ Ⓑ Ⓒ Ⓓ Ⓔ	50 Ⓐ Ⓑ Ⓒ Ⓓ Ⓔ	65 Ⓐ Ⓑ Ⓒ Ⓓ Ⓔ	80 Ⓐ Ⓑ Ⓒ Ⓓ Ⓔ
6 Ⓐ Ⓑ Ⓒ Ⓓ Ⓔ	21 Ⓐ Ⓑ Ⓒ Ⓓ Ⓔ	36 Ⓐ Ⓑ Ⓒ Ⓓ Ⓔ	51 Ⓐ Ⓑ Ⓒ Ⓓ Ⓔ	66 Ⓐ Ⓑ Ⓒ Ⓓ Ⓔ	81 Ⓐ Ⓑ Ⓒ Ⓓ Ⓔ
7 Ⓐ Ⓑ Ⓒ Ⓓ Ⓔ	22 Ⓐ Ⓑ Ⓒ Ⓓ Ⓔ	37 Ⓐ Ⓑ Ⓒ Ⓓ Ⓔ	52 Ⓐ Ⓑ Ⓒ Ⓓ Ⓔ	67 Ⓐ Ⓑ Ⓒ Ⓓ Ⓔ	82 Ⓐ Ⓑ Ⓒ Ⓓ Ⓔ
8 Ⓐ Ⓑ Ⓒ Ⓓ Ⓔ	23 Ⓐ Ⓑ Ⓒ Ⓓ Ⓔ	38 Ⓐ Ⓑ Ⓒ Ⓓ Ⓔ	53 Ⓐ Ⓑ Ⓒ Ⓓ Ⓔ	68 Ⓐ Ⓑ Ⓒ Ⓓ Ⓔ	83 Ⓐ Ⓑ Ⓒ Ⓓ Ⓔ
9 Ⓐ Ⓑ Ⓒ Ⓓ Ⓔ	24 Ⓐ Ⓑ Ⓒ Ⓓ Ⓔ	39 Ⓐ Ⓑ Ⓒ Ⓓ Ⓔ	54 Ⓐ Ⓑ Ⓒ Ⓓ Ⓔ	69 Ⓐ Ⓑ Ⓒ Ⓓ Ⓔ	84 Ⓐ Ⓑ Ⓒ Ⓓ Ⓔ
10 Ⓐ Ⓑ Ⓒ Ⓓ Ⓔ	25 Ⓐ Ⓑ Ⓒ Ⓓ Ⓔ	40 Ⓐ Ⓑ Ⓒ Ⓓ Ⓔ	55 Ⓐ Ⓑ Ⓒ Ⓓ Ⓔ	70 Ⓐ Ⓑ Ⓒ Ⓓ Ⓔ	85 Ⓐ Ⓑ Ⓒ Ⓓ Ⓔ
11 Ⓐ Ⓑ Ⓒ Ⓓ Ⓔ	26 Ⓐ Ⓑ Ⓒ Ⓓ Ⓔ	41 Ⓐ Ⓑ Ⓒ Ⓓ Ⓔ	56 Ⓐ Ⓑ Ⓒ Ⓓ Ⓔ	71 Ⓐ Ⓑ Ⓒ Ⓓ Ⓔ	86 Ⓐ Ⓑ Ⓒ Ⓓ Ⓔ
12 Ⓐ Ⓑ Ⓒ Ⓓ Ⓔ	27 Ⓐ Ⓑ Ⓒ Ⓓ Ⓔ	42 Ⓐ Ⓑ Ⓒ Ⓓ Ⓔ	57 Ⓐ Ⓑ Ⓒ Ⓓ Ⓔ	72 Ⓐ Ⓑ Ⓒ Ⓓ Ⓔ	87 Ⓐ Ⓑ Ⓒ Ⓓ Ⓔ
13 Ⓐ Ⓑ Ⓒ Ⓓ Ⓔ	28 Ⓐ Ⓑ Ⓒ Ⓓ Ⓔ	43 Ⓐ Ⓑ Ⓒ Ⓓ Ⓔ	58 Ⓐ Ⓑ Ⓒ Ⓓ Ⓔ	73 Ⓐ Ⓑ Ⓒ Ⓓ Ⓔ	88 Ⓐ Ⓑ Ⓒ Ⓓ Ⓔ
14 Ⓐ Ⓑ Ⓒ Ⓓ Ⓔ	29 Ⓐ Ⓑ Ⓒ Ⓓ Ⓔ	44 Ⓐ Ⓑ Ⓒ Ⓓ Ⓔ	59 Ⓐ Ⓑ Ⓒ Ⓓ Ⓔ	74 Ⓐ Ⓑ Ⓒ Ⓓ Ⓔ	89 Ⓐ Ⓑ Ⓒ Ⓓ Ⓔ
15 Ⓐ Ⓑ Ⓒ Ⓓ Ⓔ	30 Ⓐ Ⓑ Ⓒ Ⓓ Ⓔ	45 Ⓐ Ⓑ Ⓒ Ⓓ Ⓔ	60 Ⓐ Ⓑ Ⓒ Ⓓ Ⓔ	75 Ⓐ Ⓑ Ⓒ Ⓓ Ⓔ	90 Ⓐ Ⓑ Ⓒ Ⓓ Ⓔ

书面表达

请用黑色签字笔在答题区域内作答，超出黑色边框区域的答案无效！

样张（英语）

5

10

国家医学考试中心监制　　　　北京世纪互联软件开发有限公司设计制作　LT-1/8L 2019L146F

书 面 表 达　　　　　请用黑色签字笔在答题区域内作答，超出黑色边框区域的答案无效！

15

20

25

30

LT–1/8R 2013B002B

Hi-Fi FATMD Test 4

PAPER ONE

Part I Listening Comprehension (30%)

Section A

Directions: *In this section, you will hear fifteen short conversations between two speakers. At the end of each conversation, you will hear a question about what is said. The question will be read only once. After you hear the question, read the four possible answers marked A, B, C, and D. Choose the best answer and mark the letter of your choice on the* **ANSWER SHEET**.

Listen to the following example:

You will hear:

W: I feel faint.

M: No wonder. You haven't had a bite all day.

Question: What's the matter with the woman?

You will read:

A. She is sick.

B. She was bitten by an ant.

C. **She is hungry.**

D. She spilled her paint.

Here C is the right answer.

Sample Answer

A B ● D

Now let's begin with question Number 1.

1. A. It was called off unexpectedly.   B. It raised more money than expected.
    C. It received fewer people than expected. D. It disappointed the woman for the man's absence.

2. A. A thoracic case.   B. A nervous disorder.
    C. A stomach problem.   D. A psychiatric condition.

3. A. In the housing office on campus.   B. In the downtown hotel.
    C. At the rental agency.   D. In the nursing home.

4. A. Thrilled.   B. Refreshed.
    C. Exhausted.   D. Depressed.

5. A. To travel with his parents.   B. To organize a picnic in the country.
    C. To cruise, even without his friends.   D. To take a flight to the Maldives instead.

6. A. He's got a fever.   B. He's got nausea.
    C. He's got diarrhea.   D. He's got a runny nose.

7. A. To suture the man's wound.   B. To remove the bits of glass.
    C. To disinfect the man's wound.   D. To take a closer look at the man's wound.

8. A. Mr. Lindley had got injured.   B. Mr. Lindley had fallen asleep.
    C. Mr. Lindley had fallen off his chair.   D. Mr. Lindley had lost consciousness.

9. A. She will apply to Duke University.
    B. She will probably attend the University of Texas.
    C. She made up her mind to give up school for work.
    D. She chose Duke University over the University of Texas.

10. A. Her boyfriend broke up with her.   B. She was almost run over by a truck.
    C. One of her friends was emotionally hurt.   D. She dumped her boyfriend's truck in the river.

11. A. The patient will not accept the doctor's recommendation.
    B. The doctor lost control of the allergic reaction.
    C. The doctor finds it hard to decide what to do.
    D. The medicine is not available to the patient.

12. A. It was more expensive than the original price.   B. It was given to the woman as a gift.
    C. It was the last article on sale.   D. It was a good bargain.

13. A. Excited.   B. Impatient.
    C. Indifferent.   D. Concerned.

14. A. She regrets buying the car.   B. The car just arrived yesterday.
    C. She will certainly not buy the car.   D. This is the car she has been wanting.

15. A. He is seriously ill.   B. His work is a mess.
    C. The weather is lousy this week.   D. He has been working under pressure.

Section B

Directions: *In this part, you will hear three passages. After each one, you will hear five questions. After each question, read the four possible answers marked A, B, C, and D. Choose the best answer and mark the letter of your choice on the* **ANSWER SHEET**.

Sample Answer
A B ● D

Passage One

16. A. He has got bowel cancer.   B. He has got heart disease.
    C. He has got bone cancer.   D. He has got heartburn.

17. A. To have a colonoscopy.   B. To seek a second opinion.
    C. To be put on chemotherapy.   D. To have his bowel removed.

18. A. A pretty minor surgery.   B. A normal life ahead of him.
    C. A miracle in his coming years.   D. A life without any inconveniences.

19. A. Thankful.   B. Admiring.
    C. Resentful.   D. Respectful.

20. A. It was based on the symptoms the man had described.
    B. It was prescribed considering possible complications.
    C. It was given according to the man's actual condition.
    D. It was effective because of a proper intervention.

Passage Two

21. A. Smoking and lung cancer.   B. Lung cancer and the sexes.
    C. How to quit smoking.   D. How to prevent lung cancer.

22. A. Current smokers exclusively.   B. Second-hand smokers.

C. With a lung problem.　　D. At age 40 or over.

23. A. 156.　　B. 269.
    C. 7,498.　　D. 9,427.
24. A. Smoking is the culprit in causing lung cancer.
    B. Women are more vulnerable to lung cancer than men.
    C. Women are found to be more addicted to smoking than men.
    D. When struck by lung cancer, men seem to live longer than women.
25. A. Lung cancer can be early detected.
    B. Lung cancer is deadly but preventable.
    C. Lung cancer is fatal and unpredictable.
    D. Smoking affects the lungs of men and women differently.

Passage Three
26. A. A hobby.　　B. The whole world.
    C. A learning experience.　　D. A career to earn a living.
27. A. Her legs were broken.　　B. Her arms were broken.
    C. Her shoulders were severely injured.　　D. Her cervical vertebrae were seriously injured.
28. A. She learned a foreign language.　　B. She learned to make friends.
    C. She learned to be a teacher.　　D. She learned living skills.
29. A. She worked as skiing coach.　　B. She was a college instructor.
    C. She was a social worker in the clinic.　　D. She worked as elementary school teacher.
30. A. Optimistic and hard-bitten.　　B. Pessimistic and cynical.
    C. Humorous and funny.　　D. Kind and reliable.

Part Ⅱ Vocabulary (10%)

Section A

Directions: *In this section, all the statements are incomplete, beneath each of which are four words or phrases marked A, B, C, and D. Choose the word or phrase that can best complete the statement and mark the letter of your choice on the* **ANSWER SHEET**.

31. I am afraid that you'll have to _____ the deterioration of the condition.
    A. account for　　B. call for
    C. look for　　D. make for
32. Twelve hours a week seemed a generous _____ of your time to the nursing home.
    A. affliction　　B. alternative
    C. allocation　　D. alliance
33. Every product is _____ tested before being put into the market.
    A. expensively　　B. exceptionally
    C. exhaustively　　D. exclusively
34. Having clean hands is one of the _____ rules when preparing food.
    A. potent　　B. conditional
    C. inseparable　　D. cardinal
35. The educators should try hard to develop the _____ abilities of children.
    A. cohesive　　B. cognitive

C. collective   D. comic

36. Mortgage _____ had risen in the last year because the number of low-income families was on the increase.

    A. defects   B. deficits
    C. defaults   D. deceptions

37. The symptoms may be _____ by certain drugs.

    A. exaggerated   B. exacerbated
    C. exceeded   D. exhibited

38. Her story was a complete _____ from start to finish, so nobody believed in her.

    A. facility   B. fascination
    C. fabrication   D. faculty

39. The police investigating the traffic accident have not ruled out _____.

    A. salvage   B. safeguard
    C. sabotage   D. sacrifice

40. The government always _____ on the background of employees who are hired for sensitive military projects.

    A. takes up   B. checks up
    C. works out   D. looks into

Section B

Directions: *In this section, each of the following sentences has a word or phrase underlined, beneath which are four words or phrases. Choose the word or phrase which can best keep the meaning of the original sentence if it is substituted for the underlined part. Then mark your choice on the* **ANSWER SHEET.**

41. The 19th century physiology was dominated by the study of the transformations of food energy into body mass and activity.

    A. boosted   B. governed
    C. clarified   D. pioneered

42. Surely, it would be sensible to get a second opinion before taking any further action.

    A. realistic   B. sensitive
    C. reasonable   D. sensational

43. The Chinese people hold their ancestors in great veneration.

    A. recognition   B. sincerity
    C. heritage   D. honour

44. I worked to develop the requisite skill for a managerial.

    A. perfect   B. exquisite
    C. unique   D. necessary

45. If exercise is a bodily maintenance activity and an index of physiological age, the lack of sufficient exercise may either cause or hasten aging.

    A. instance   B. indicator
    C. appearance   D. option

46. The doctor advised Ken to avoid strenuous exercise.

    A. arduous   B. demanding
    C. potent   D. continuous

47. The hospital should be held <u>accountable</u> for the quality of care it delivers.
    A. practicable
    B. reliable
    C. flexible
    D. responsible

48. Greenpeace has been invited to <u>appraise</u> the environment costs of such an operation.
    A. esteem
    B. appreciate
    C. evaluate
    D. approve

49. The company still hopes to find a buyer, but the future looks <u>bleak</u>.
    A. chilly
    B. dismal
    C. promising
    D. fanatic

50. These were vital decisions that <u>bore upon</u> the happiness of everybody.
    A. ensured
    B. ruined
    C. achieved
    D. influenced

Part III　Cloze (10%)

Directions: *In this section, there is a passage with ten numbered blanks. For each blank, there are four choices marked A, B, C, and D listed on the right side. Choose the best answer and mark the letter of your choice on the* **ANSWER SHEET**.

Are some people born clever and others born stupid? Or is intelligence developed by our environment and our experiences? Strangely __51__ , the answer to both these questions is yes. To some extent, our intelligence is given us at birth, and no amount of special education can make a genius __52__ a child born with low intelligence. On the other hand, a child who lives in a boring environment will develop his intelligence less than the one who lives in rich and varied surroundings. Thus the __53__ of a person's intelligence are fixed at birth, but whether or not he reaches those limits will depend on his __54__ . This view, not held by most experts, can be supported in a number of ways.

It is easy to show that intelligence is to some extent __55__ we are born with. The closer the blood relationship between two people, the closer they are likely to be in intelligence. Thus if we take two unrelated people __56__ , it is likely that their degrees of intelligence will be completely different. If on the other hand we take two identical twins they will likely be as intelligent as each other. Relations like brothers and sisters, parents and children, usually have __57__ intelligence, and this clearly suggests that intelligence depends on birth.

__58__ now that we take identical twins and put them in different environments. We might send one, for

51. A. quite
    B. enough
    C. sure
    D. so

52. A. out of
    B. into
    C. from within
    D. off

53. A. amounts
    B. qualities
    C. limits
    D. scores

54. A. disposition
    B. perception
    C. endowment
    D. environment

55. A. anything
    B. something
    C. nothing
    D. everything

56. A. in advance
    B. for effect
    C. at random
    D. under way

57. A. similar
    B. various
    C. appropriate
    D. inborn

58. A. Look
    B. Believe
    C. Suggest
    D. Imagine

example, to a university and the other to a factory where the work is boring. We would soon find differences in intelligence developing, and this indicates that environment __59__ birth plays a part. This conclusion is also suggested by the __60__ that people who live in close contact with each other, but who are not related at all, are likely to have similar degrees of intelligence.

59. A. and   B. or rather
    C. as well as   D. but for

60. A. fact   B. event
    C. condition   D. environment

Part Ⅳ   Reading Comprehension (30%)

Directions: *In this part there are six passages, each of which is followed by five questions. For each question there are four possible answers marked A, B, C, and D. Choose the best answer and mark the letter of your choice on the* **ANSWER SHEET**.

Passage One

Fourteen-year-old Sean MeCallum lay in a hospital bed waiting for a new heart. Without it, Sean would die. Sean's case is not unusual. Everyday many people die because there just aren't enough human organs to go around.

Now scientists say they can alter the genetic make-up of certain animals so that their organs may be acceptable to humans. With this gene-altering technique to overcome our immune rejection to foreign organs, scientists hope to use pig hearts for transplants by the year 2008.

That prospect, however, has stirred up strong opposition among animal fight activists. They protest that the whole idea of using animal organs is cruel and unjust. Some scientists also fear such transplants may transmit unknown diseases to humans.

Others believe transplanting animal organs into humans is unnecessary. Millions of dollars spent on breeding pigs for their organs could be better spent on health education programs. They believe seventy-five percent of the heart disease cases that lead to a need for organ transplant are preventable. The key is to convince people to eat healthfully, and not to smoke or drink alcohol. Scientists could also use research funds to improve artificial organs.

Still others believe that though new inventions and prevention programs may help, spending money to encourage more people to donate their organs is an even better idea. If enough people were educated about organ donations, everyone who needed an organ could be taken off the waiting list in a year.

61. What is the problem the passage begins with?

    A. A high mortality rate of immune rejection.

    B. A malpractice in heart transplantation.

    C. An unusual case of organ transplant.

    D. A shortage of human organs.

62. Not only is the gene-altering technique a technical issue, according to the passage, but also it _____.

    A. introduces an issue of inhumanity

    B. raises the issue of justice in medicine

    C. presents a significant threat to the human nature

    D. pushes the practice of organ transplant to the limits

63. Doubtful of the necessity of using animal organs, some scientists _____.

    A. are to narrow the scope of organ transplants

    B. switch to the development of artificial organs

    C. come up with alternatives to the current problem

    D. set out to pursue better ways of treating heart disease

64. It can be inferred from the concluding paragraph of the passage that _____.

    A. the gene-altering technique will help those waiting for organ transplants

    B. the present supply of human organs still has potential to be explored

    C. people prefer the use of animal organs for medical purposes

    D. the gene-altering technique leaves much to be desired

65. The information the passage carries is _____.

    A. enlightening   B. unbelievable

    C. imaginative   D. factual

Passage Two

Here is a great irony of 21st-century global health: While many hundreds of millions of people lack adequate food as a result of economic inequities, political corruption, or warfare, many hundreds of millions more are overweight to the point of increased risk for diet-related chronic diseases. Obesity is a worldwide phenomenon, affecting children as well as adults and forcing all but the poorest countries to divert scarce resources away from food security to take care of people with preventable heart disease and diabetes.

To reverse the obesity epidemic, we must address the fundamental cause. Overweight comes from consuming more food energy than is expended in activity. The cause of this imbalance also is ironic: improved prosperity. People use extra income to eat more and be less physically active. Market economies encourage this. They turn people with expendable income into consumers of aggressively marketed foods that are high in energy but low in nutritional value, and of cars, televisions sets, and computers that promote sedentary behavior. Gaining weight is good business. Food is particularly big business because everyone eats.

Moreover, food is so overproduced that many countries, especially the rich ones, have far more than they need—another irony. In the United States, to take an extreme example, most adults—of all ages, incomes, educational levels, and census categories—are overweight. The U.S. food supply provides 3,800 kilocalories per person per day, nearly twice as much as required by many adults. Overabundant food forces companies to compete for sales through advertising, health claims, new products, larger portions, and campaigns directed toward children. Food marketing promotes weight gain. Indeed, it is difficult to think of any major industry that might benefit if people ate less food; certainly not the agriculture, food product, grocery, restaurant, diet, or drug industries. All flourish when people eat more, and all employ armies of lobbyists to discourage governments from doing anything to inhibit overeating.

66. The great irony of 21st-century global public health refers to _____.

    A. the cause of obesity and its counteractive measures

    B. the insufficient and superfluous consumption of food

    C. the scarce natural resource and the negligence of food security

    D. the consumption of food and the increased risk for diet-related diseases

67. To address the fundamental cause of the obesity epidemic, according to the passage, is_____.

    A. to improve political and economic management

    B. to cope with the energy imbalance issue

    C. to combat diet-related chronic diseases

    D. to increase investment in global health

68. As we can learn from the passage, the second irony refers to _____.

    A. affluence and obesity

    B. food energy and nutritional value

    C. food business and economic prosperity

D. diseases of civilization and pathology of inactivity

69. As a result of the third irony, people _____.

    A. consume 3,800 kilocalories on a daily basis   B. complain about food overproduction

    C. have to raise their food expenses   D. are driven towards weight gain

70. Which of the following can be excluded as we can understand based on the passage?

    A. The economic dimension.   B. The political dimension.

    C. The humane dimension.   D. The dietary dimension.

Passage Three

Women find a masculine face with a large jaw and a prominent brow—more attractive when they are most likely to conceive, according to a study published in the June 24 *NATURE*. Before, during, and just after menstruation, however, they seem to be drawn to less angular, more "feminine" male faces, the researchers report.

"Other studies of female preference, mainly for odors, show changes across the menstrual cycle," says lead author Ian Penton-Voak of the University of St. Andrews in Scotland. "We thought it would be interesting to look at visual preferences and see if they changed also."

The researchers showed 39 Japanese women composite male faces that emphasized masculine or feminine facial features to differing degrees. The women preferred images with more masculine features when they were in the fertile phase of their menses but favored more feminine features during their less fertile phase.

The type of face women find attractive also seems to depend on the kind of relationship they wish to pursue, according to another experiment.

The cyclic preference for masculine faces was evident among 23 British women asked to choose the most attractive face for a short-term relationship, Penton-Voak says. The 26 women asked to choose an attractive face for a long-term relationship, however, preferred the more feminine features throughout their menstrual cycle.

Another 22 women who were using oral contraceptives did not show monthly changes in the faces they preferred even for short-term relationships, indicating that hormones might play a role in determining attractiveness, Penton-Voak says.

Men whose faces have some feminine softness are perceived as "kinder" men who may make better husbands and partners, he adds, while macho features may be associated with higher testosterone（睾丸素）levels and good genes. He cautions, however, that research hasn't yet shown a link between a woman's preferences in such tests and her actual behavior.

71. The researchers made a study on _____.

    A. women's menstrual cycle   B. men's preferred female images

    C. women's visual preferences of men   D. men's masculine and feminine features

72. Women are drawn to a masculine face, according to the researchers, when they _____.

    A. grow to be more feminine   B. are on oral contraceptives

    C. are ready for conception   D. are on menstruation

73. It was found in Britain that women's preferred male images were influenced by _____.

    A. their family planning   B. the years of marriage they had

    C. the length of their menstrual cycle   D. the term of a relationship they seek

74. Just because the studies of female preferences show changes across the menstrual cycle, as Penton-Voak implies, does not mean that _____.

    A. visual preferences do exist   B. a woman acts this way in reality

C. a man will buy into the phenomenon   D. men and women prefer the same image

75. Which of the following can be the best title for the passage?

    A. Does a woman judge from a man's appearance?

    B. Is there such a thing as beauty in the world?

    C. Are women more emotional than men?

    D. Is beauty more than meets the eye?

Passage Four

WELL—do they or don't they? For years, controversy has raged over whether the electromagnetic fields produced by power lines could cause cancer, especially leukaemia in young children. But in Britain last week, confusion reached new heights.

One team from Bristol announced that it had evidence to back a controversial but plausible theory which would explain how power lines might cause cancer (electric fields attract airborne pollutants). Only to be followed by the release of results by another group in London which suggested there is nothing to worry about. What is going on?

Actually, the confusion may be more apparent than real. There can be no doubt that the effects of power lines on water droplets, pollutants and naturally occurring radon uncovered by the Bristol team are real and interesting. But to suggest that they have anything to do with leukaemia in children is premature. The extra exposure to pollution for a child living near power lines would be tiny, and it is not obvious why radon—a gas normally associated with lung cancer—would cause leukaemia in children.

The second study, which drew reassuring blank, is the world's biggest ever probe of the statistical link between childhood cancers and magnetic fields of the sort produced by power lines and electrical appliances. It is one of several recent studies that have failed to find a link.

Unlike earlier research, these newer studies involved going into homes to measure the electromagnetic fields. The fields they measured included input from major power lines if they were nearby.

Which is not to say the research is perfect. Critics argue that Britain's childhood cancer study, for example, has not yet taken into account the surges in exposure that might come from, say, switching appliances on and off. And some people might wonder why measurements of the electric fields that are also produced by power lines did not figure in last week's study. But neither criticism amounts to a fatal blow. Electrical fields cannot penetrate the body significantly, for example.

A more serious concern is whether the British research provides an all-clear signal for such countries as the US where power lines carry more current and therefore produce higher magnetic fields. Pedants（书呆子）would conclude that it doesn't. But these countries will not have long to wait for answers from a major Japanese study.

In Britain, the latest epidemiological study can be taken as the final word on the matter. If the electromagnetic fields in British homes can in some unforeseen way increase the risk of cancer, we can now be as certain as science allows that the increase is too tiny to measure.

76. Both the question "Well—do they or don't they?" and the question "What is going on?" suggest _____.

    A. the high incidence of leukaemia

    B. the advent of bewilderment among people

    C. the warning of the worsening air pollution

    D. the tense relation between Bristol and London

77. What would the author say of the results of the first study?

    A. Enlightening.   B. Insignificant.

C. Reassuring.   D. Apparent.

78. What can be suggested from the results of the second study?

    A. There does exist a danger zone near power lines.

    B. There is much to be improved in terms of design.

    C. There is nothing to worry about as to power lines.

    D. There is no link between the first and second study.

79. It can be inferred from the passage that the British outcomes _____.

    A. are expected to convince nobody but pedants

    B. were found to have left much room for doubt

    C. could have implications in such countries as the US

    D. will be consistent with the Japanese ones in the near future

80. To conclude, the author _____.

    A. reassures us of the reliability of the latest research in Britain

    B. asks for improved measurements for such an investigation

    C. points out the drawbacks of the latest research in Britain

    D. urges further investigations on the issue

Passage Five

Smoking causes wrinkles by upsetting the body's mechanism for renewing skin, say scientists in Japan. Dermatologists say the finding confirms the long-held view that smoking ages skin prematurely.

Skin stays healthy and young-looking because of a fine balance between two processes that are constantly at work. The first breaks down old skin while the second makes new skin. The body breaks down the old skin with enzymes called matrix metalloproteinases, or MMPs. They chop up the fibers that form collagen（胶原质）—the connective tissue that makes up around 80 percent of normal skin.

Akimichi Morita and his colleagues at Nagoya City University Medical School suspected that smoking disrupted the body's natural process of breaking down old skin and renewing it. To test their idea, they first made a solution of cigarette smoke by pumping smoke through a saline（盐的）solution. Smoke was sucked from cigarettes for two seconds every minute. Tiny drops of this smoke solution were added to dishes of human fibroblasts, the skin cells that produce collagen.

After a day in contact with smoke solution, the researchers tested the skin cells to see how much collagen-degrading MMP they were making. Morita found that cells exposed to cigarette smoke had produced far more MMP than normal skin cells.

Morita also tested the skin cells to see how much new collagen they were producing. He found that the smoke caused a drop in the production of fresh collagen by up to 40 percent.

He says that this combined effect of degrading collagen more rapidly and producing less new collagen is probably what causes premature skin ageing in smokers. In both cases, the more concentrated the smoke solution the greater the effect on collagen. "This suggests the amount of collagen is important for skin ageing," he says. "It looks like less collagen means more wrinkle formation".

Morita doesn't know if this is the whole story of why smokers have more wrinkles. But he plans to confirm his findings by testing skin samples from smokers and non-smokers of various ages to see if the smoking has the same effect on collagen. "So far we've only done this in the lab," he says. "We don't know exactly what happens in the body yet—that might take some time."

Other dermatologists are impressed by the work. "This is fascinating," says Lawrence Parish, director of the Centre for International Dermatology at Thomas Jefferson University Hospital in Philadelphia. This confirms scientifically what we've long expected, he says. "Tobacco smoke is injurious to skin."

81. Healthy skin lies in _____.

    A. a well-kept balance between two working processes

    B. the two processes of breaking down skin cells

    C. a fine balance in the number of cigarettes

    D. the two steps of forming collagen

82. For the Japanese scientists, to test their idea is _____.

    A. to verify the aging of human beings

    B. to find out the mechanism of renewing skin

    C. to prove the two processes of wrinkle formation

    D. to confirm the hazards of smoking proven otherwise

83. The Japanese scientists tested their idea using _____.

    A. MMPs to form fresh collagen   B. cigarette smoke to contaminate skin cells

    C. human fibroblasts to produce fresh collagen   D. non-smokers to be exposed to cigarette smoke

84. As inferred from Morita's results, smoking _____.

    A. could stimulate the production of fresh collagen

    B. is unlikely to promote the production of MMP

    C. tends to cause skin to age prematurely

    D. may cause collagen to die by 60%

85. Morita implies that his findings _____.

    A. took less time than expected   B. were hard to accept in dermatology

    C. were not exclusively based on the lab   D. need to be further verified in the human body

Passage Six

Today, I sit in a surgical ICU beside my favorite Jack as he recovers from a five-hour operation to repair a massive aortic aneurysm. For me it has been a journey into the medical system as an inexperienced consumer rather than in my usual position as a seasoned provider. This journey to an urban referral center has produced some disappointing surprises for Dad, and especially for me. For the past two days, my beloved Jack has been called "Harold" (his first name; Jack is his middle name). Of course, there is nothing wrong with "Harold"—it was what he was called in the army—but Dad never has been "Harold", except to those who really don't know him. Telephone callers at our family home who asked for "Harold" were always red flags that the caller was a telemarketer or insurance salesperson.

Dad doesn't correct his physicians or the office receptionists—he is from the old school, where it is impolite to question or correct your physician. Once he was an almost ideal "Jack", strong, athletic, quietly confident, and imminently trustworthy, but his recent renal failure and dialysis treatments, his stroke and his constant tremor have robbed him of his strength, mobility, and golf game, but not of his will or love of his family. Part of the reason he agreed to undertake this risky operation at his advanced age was because his wife and sisters still need his protective support. With so much at risk, he faced this life-threatening challenge in a city far away from his home and friends and in a place where he is greeted as "Harold".

86. The author relates the story _____.

    A. from a consumer's point of view

    B. with a view to punctuating patient rights

    C. according to his own standards of health care

    D. based on his own unpleasant medical treatment

87. Apparently, the author's father _____.
    A. did not like to be called by the first name B. was not well taken care of as expected
    C. was mistaken for somebody else D. was treated like a businessman

88. As the author implies, his father _____.
    A. encountered so many impolite physicians B. did nothing but kept quiet in the hospital
    C. accepted the way he was greeted D. had his diagnosis made wrongly

89. What the story implies is that _____.
    A. people are what they are called
    B. nobody likes to be called Harold in English
    C. a patient should be called as he or she wishes
    D. a patient cannot be called by the first name in the hospital

90. The author describes his "Jack" in a tone of _____.
    A. admiration B. inspiration
    C. indignation D. expectation

GO TO THE NEXT PAGE FOR PAPER TWO: WRITING.

PAPER TWO

Part Ⅴ　Writing (20%)

Directions: *In this part there is an essay in Chinese. Read it carefully and then write a summary of 200 words in English on the **ANSWER SHEET**. Make sure that your summary covers the major points of the essay.*

答题要求

（1）紧扣主题，归纳总结；

（2）涵盖所有重要内容；

（3）避免选择原句进行简单翻译；

（4）无须推演或推论。

珍爱生命从护心开始

生命第一杀手

这些年来，随着我国经济的发展，在人们解决了温饱之后，伴随而来的是与吸烟、缺乏运动、紧张和过度饮食等不良生活方式相关的慢性疾病，尤其是心血管疾病、肿瘤等已经成为危害健康、危及生命的第一杀手。

近年来，"猝死"事件在各地屡有发生。压力过大，劳累过度，使得不少中青年长期处于亚健康状态，积重难返而猝死。在众多猝死事件中，多数是由心肌梗死引起的。而半数以上的心肌梗死是没有先兆的，突然发病，致死或致残；在心肌梗死发病早期死亡者中，半数都死于到达医院之前。

在很多人的印象里，高血压、冠心病、心肌梗死好像是中老年人的"专利"，其实不然，现在每天医院急诊室、监护室里都能看到一些非常年轻的心肌梗死患者，而且越来越多。

无知者"无畏"

很多人并不是死于无钱，而是死于无知，即缺乏预防意识，缺乏对健康的忧患意识，这在"白骨精"（白领、骨干、精英）中尤为突出。他们白天忙于工作，晚上忙于应酬，很少有人把自己的健康放在心上。

20 世纪 50 年代出生的这一代人，更多地受益于经济发展所带来的便捷、舒适的生活，这种生活方式使得他们中的一部分人已经成为目前高血压、糖尿病和肥胖流行的"主力军"。但是，国内外大量的医学研究表明，吸烟，高热量、高脂肪饮食摄入过多，运动量减少等不健康生活方式，正在成为引发包括心肌梗死在内的各种心血管疾病的"催化剂"。正是由于这些危险因素没有被认识，没有得到很好的重视和控制，才使得情况变得越来越糟。

值得注意的是，不健康的生活方式所致的心血管疾病多是"隐性杀手"，平时无明显症状，但却在不知不觉中残害人们的健康。历经几年、十几年、甚至数十年的"沉默"，在毫无症状或先兆的情况下，以突然发病的形式瞬间结束人们的生命。相当多的病人第一次发病或第一次有临床表现就是心肌梗死，甚至猝死进而结束生命。

令人担忧的是，现在很多"白骨精"们根本意识不到自己是心血管疾病的高危人群，甚至幻想患病以后再亡羊补牢。实际上，在长期的超负荷"压迫"下，他们一旦发病就会一发而不可收拾，第一次就往往可能是猝死，所以一定不能心存侥幸。

管住嘴　迈开腿

血脂的异常和胆固醇升高、吸烟、糖尿病、高血压、中心性肥胖、日常生活缺乏运动、饮食缺乏蔬菜水果、紧张的情绪都已经被证明是诱发心血管疾病的重要危险因素，既然我们已经知道心血管疾病是一个多重危险因子的疾病，那么应首先从预防危险因素上做起，而不要等到患了高血压再去吃降压药物，得了血脂高再去降血脂。

心血管疾病是可防、可控、可救的。吸烟是万恶之源，不只是危害心血管，也是引起呼吸系统和多种癌症的"罪犯"。吸烟害己更害人，吸烟不是"嗜好"，而是疾病。肥胖和血脂异常也可明显增加高血压、心肌梗死等的危险。

心血管防治要注重"治未病"，对每一个人来说，要有一个健康的身体，先要不吸烟，"管住嘴"，"迈开腿"。特别要从青少年抓起，引导青少年从小养成健康文明的生活习惯，告别烟草，告别垃圾食品，热爱和坚持运动，保持良好的体重。

"迈开腿"，除了爬山、游泳等运动以外，要把路走起来。现在很多人都自觉或不自觉地开始慢慢地在变"懒"，能不动就不动，特别是有的青年人，进门就找电梯，出门就打的，为什么不能进门先找楼梯走一走呢？如果大家能坚持每天快步走一万步的路，持之以恒，定将受益匪浅。饭吃八成饱，日行万步路，为最有效的减肥方法。

THIS IS THE END OF THIS OFFICIAL TEST.

Hi-Fi FATMD Test 4
Answer Keys
（非标准答案，仅供参考）

Part Ⅰ. Listening

1-3: CCA   4-6: CCC   7-9: ADB   10-12: ACD   13-15: BCD   16-18: ADB   19-21: CAA

22-24: DBA   25-27: BBD   28-30: DDA

Part Ⅱ. Vocabulary

31-35: CCCDB   36-40: CBCCB   41-45: BCDDB   46-50: BDCBD

Part Ⅲ. Cloze

51-55: BACDB   56-60: CADCA

Part Ⅳ. Reading

61-65: DACBD   66-70: BBADC   71-75: CCDBA   76-80: BBCDA   81-85: ADBCD

86-90: AACCA

Part Ⅴ. Writing

Prevention of Cardiovascular Diseases

1. No. 1 killer

In recent years, chronic diseases, especially cardiovascular diseases, tumors, etc., have become the major cause/No.1 killer to people's lives. Many deaths are sudden deaths because of myocardial infarction. The infarction was induced by prolonged chronic subhealth. Obviously, a heart attack is prevalent in this aspect.

2. Poor awareness of care for the heart

Many people died of a lack of awareness of healthcare for the heart rather than poverty. Many white-collar workers are too busy to take good care of their hearts, which results in a heart attack or infarction. Besides, due to improved standard of living, many modern people suffer from sub-health because of unhealthy lifestyles and habits such as overeating, drinking, over-intake of high-fat and high-heat foods and lack of physical exercise. All this may cause cardiovascular diseases.

3. How to prevent heart attack/infarction?

As it has been proved, unhealthy eating and living habits are the culprits of subhealth. So, the best ways to prevent this include eating less and doing more exercise. This suggests that we should stop smoking and live a more active lifestyle.

Conclusively, cardiovascular diseases are dangerous but not unpreventable if we live in a healthy way.

Tapescript for the Listening Comprehension

Section A

1. W: How many people turned up at the fund-raising event?

   M: Fewer people came than we had expected. It was disappointing, for we made a little money for the art organization.

   W: Sorry. I wasn't able to attend. I intended to.

   M: What did the man say about the fund-raising event?   C)

2. M: The refluxes are often caused by the relaxation of the sphincter which opens at the wrong time, allowing the contents to flow into the flow of the oesophagus. What do you think of the results?

    W: It burns. That's cause of the heart burn, right?

    M: What are they talking about?   C)

3. W: Excuse me. I understand that this office helps students with housing. Is that right?

    M: Are you a student in the nursing program? May I see your ID card? ...mm. Yes, we can certainly help you. Where are you staying now?

    W: I just arrived yesterday. I'm staying at the hotel across the street.

    M: Or will you be living alone or do you have a family? Or would you be interested in sharing housing?

    W: Where does the conversation most probably take place?   A)

4. M: Let's call it a day. We've been active for hours.

    W: I'm beat too. Let's get something to eat.

    M: We will be able to feel better with a little nutrition.

    W: How are these speakers feeling?   C)

5. W: I heard that you and some friends are organizing a cruise to Maldives.

    M: It never really got off the ground.

    W: That's too bad. It sounded like fun.

    M: Yeah. I'm still planning to go. Alone if I have to.

    W: What is the man planning to do?   C)

6. M: Doc. I'm afraid I have to run.

    W: Are you going to the toilet often?

    M: Haven't stopped since very early in the morning.

    W: What did you have for breakfast?

    M: Just cereal and a few cups of tea.

    W: What is the man's problem?   C)

7. W: Take off your shirt and I will take a closer look.

    M: Can you see any bits of glass?

    W: Yes, I've removed them all and disinfected the wound. The next thing I shall do is to stitch you up.

    M: What is the woman going to do next?   A)

8. M: Hello, Dr. Calvin here. What seems to be the problem?

    W: It's Mr. Lindley. I found him in his chair, white as a sheet. I thought he passed out.

    M: What can we learn from the conversation?   D)

9. W: Jackie is considering attending the University of Texas in Houston.

    M: Really? I thought she was registered at Duke University.

    W: That's true. But she decided she didn't want to be so far from home.

    M: What does the woman say about Jackie?   B)

10. M: My gosh. You look like you've got a run-over by a truck. What's wrong?

    W: My boyfriend just dumped me for another girl.

    M: What does the woman mean?   A)

11. M: The only medicine that will save the patient's leg produces a series of allergic reaction.

    W: The doctor is between a rock and a hard place now?

    M: What does the woman imply?   C)

12. W: Did you like the Chanel bag that I got?

M: You must have a rich boyfriend because that bag is so expensive.

W: I bought it on Ebay. It was only 1/10th of the original price. And purchase online was so easy.

M: What is said about the Chanel bag? D)

13. W: Bring some medicine when you go to picnic. Insects can transmit disease.

M: I see. You've said that several times.

W: Which of the following can best describe the man's feeling? B)

14. M: Please look at this car. It's nice.

W: This car has a lot of faults. You must think I was born yesterday if you expect me to buy it.

M: What does the woman mean? C)

15. W: How are you doing these days with your new job?

M: Not very well, I'm afraid. I'm feeling lousy.

W: Really? Why?

M: It's been a tense week.

W: What does the man mean? D)

Section B

Passage One

W: Well, you'll probably have to have an operation to remove the bowel or some of it. It's too diseased to save, I'm afraid.

M: How will I go on without a bowel? How can I live without a bowel?

W: During the operation, they will fit you externally with a colostomy bag.

M: You mean a bag of shit hanging inside my clothes?

W: Well, that's perhaps an unnecessarily crude way of putting it. But broadly speaking, yes. It is sealed and odour-free. They'll show you how to empty it and change it for yourself. And nobody need ever know you've got one unless you tell them.

M: Well, thanks a lot. Cancer of the bowel. All this time you have been prescribing me tablets for heart burn. And it turns out I've got a cancer of the bowel? Oh, thanks a million. What next? How will I go on now? Will I be able to live any kind of normal life? Tell me.

W: I prescribed for you on the basis of the symptoms you yourself described to me. Only a colonoscopy could reveal your condition. No doctor could diagnose your condition without the hospital test that I arranged for you. And yes, you will be able to lead a pretty normal life and go work and everything. Nobody need ever know a thing unless you choose to tell them. And you've a full life ahead of you.

16. What is wrong with the man? A)

17. What does the doctor recommend the man to do? D)

18. What does the doctor assure the man of ? B)

19. What is the man's attitude toward the doctor? C)

20. What does the doctor say about the previous treatment for the patient? A)

Passage Two

For years, researchers have debated whether smoking affects the lungs of men and women differently. And in the most compelling studies on the topic to date, researchers are determined that women are as twice vulnerable to lung cancer as men. But in a surprising twist, they die at half the rate of men. The study, which was published last week in the Journal of American Medical Association（JAMA）, included 9,427 men and 7,498 women from throughout the north America who were healthy, at least 40 years old, and either current or former smokers. Over the course of more than eight years, a group of investigators led by Doctor Claudia

Hemshky of the Wile Medical College of New York City identified lung tumours in 113 of the men and 156 of the women. Then the researchers kept track of who lived and for how long as well as the treatment the participants were given. The studies show that both sexes tended to be in their late sixties when they received the lung cancer diagnosis but that the women usually had smoked considerably less than the men. Still at each stage of lung cancer, the women lived longer than the men. If the reported results are confirmed, there are a few hints from other researches that might explain the sex difference.

Women's bodies appear to have greater difficulty repairing the damage to the genes caused by smoking. But there is also some evidence that estrogen which is found in women's lungs as well as their ovaries may interfere with some tumours' ability to grow. There is one thing about which all investigators already agree: lung cancer is particularly deadly and almost entirely preventable, so the take-home message is clear—Don't smoke. And if you do smoke, quit!

21. What is the talk mainly about?　　A)
22. What was one of the requirements to the participants of the study?　　D)
23. Over the course of more than eight years, how many of the participants developed lung cancer?　　B)
24. Which of the following is one finding of the study?　　A)
25. What is the consensus among all the investigators on smoking?　　B)

Passage Three

Joe was an average skiier, competing and winning numerous titles in junior and senior national ski events. As Joe says, "Skiing was it, everything, my world." Joe's world collapsed on January 30th, 1955 when she skiied off the outer round and landed helplessly on the slope. Her fourth, fifth and sixth cervical vertebraes were broken. For days, Joe hovered between life and death. By April it became clear that she would be paralyzed from the shoulders down. Joe underwent rehabilitation therapy with cheerful determination. She learned to write, to type and to feed herself. Once she had mastered daily living skills, she enrolled in a university in California at Los Angeles, where she studied art, German and English. After overcoming yet another personal tragedy（悲剧），the death of her boyfriend in a plane crash, Joe graduated in 1961. By this time, Joe had chosen a new career goal, teaching elementary school children. Officials at UCLA, however, rejected her application for admission to the graduate school of education because of her paralysis. But she persevered working with children in the UCLA clinic school. When her family moved to Seattle, Joe's able to fulfil her new dream. She attended to the school of education at University of Washington and began her new life's work as a teacher. She taught school first in Washington, then Beverly Hill, California, finally moved back to Beshet in 1975 when she taught special education in Beshet Union Elementary School until her retirement in 1996.

26. What did ski mean to Joe before the accident?　　B)
27. What happened to Joe when she skiied off the outer round?　　D)
28. What did Joe learn during her rehabilitation?　　D)
29. What did Joe do as her new career?　　D)
30. What is the most impressive about Joe's personality?　　A)

Hi-Fi FATMD Test 5

国家医学考试中心标准答题卡

姓　名

准考证号

报考学校

考生须知

1.答题前，考生务必用黑色字迹签字笔或水笔将姓名、准考证号、报考学校填写清楚。

2.按照题号顺序在各题目的答题区域内作答，未在对应的答题区域作答或超出答题区域的作答均不给分。

3.选择题用2B铅笔作答，不得使用涂改液。

条形码粘贴框

填涂说明　　正确填涂 ●　　错误填涂 ⊘ ⊗ ⊙ ⊖

缺考违纪标记栏：　缺考 ○　　作弊 ○　　（此项由监考人员填涂！）

选择题

1 Ⓐ Ⓑ Ⓒ Ⓓ Ⓔ	16 Ⓐ Ⓑ Ⓒ Ⓓ Ⓔ	31 Ⓐ Ⓑ Ⓒ Ⓓ Ⓔ	46 Ⓐ Ⓑ Ⓒ Ⓓ Ⓔ	61 Ⓐ Ⓑ Ⓒ Ⓓ Ⓔ	76 Ⓐ Ⓑ Ⓒ Ⓓ Ⓔ
2 Ⓐ Ⓑ Ⓒ Ⓓ Ⓔ	17 Ⓐ Ⓑ Ⓒ Ⓓ Ⓔ	32 Ⓐ Ⓑ Ⓒ Ⓓ Ⓔ	47 Ⓐ Ⓑ Ⓒ Ⓓ Ⓔ	62 Ⓐ Ⓑ Ⓒ Ⓓ Ⓔ	77 Ⓐ Ⓑ Ⓒ Ⓓ Ⓔ
3 Ⓐ Ⓑ Ⓒ Ⓓ Ⓔ	18 Ⓐ Ⓑ Ⓒ Ⓓ Ⓔ	33 Ⓐ Ⓑ Ⓒ Ⓓ Ⓔ	48 Ⓐ Ⓑ Ⓒ Ⓓ Ⓔ	63 Ⓐ Ⓑ Ⓒ Ⓓ Ⓔ	78 Ⓐ Ⓑ Ⓒ Ⓓ Ⓔ
4 Ⓐ Ⓑ Ⓒ Ⓓ Ⓔ	19 Ⓐ Ⓑ Ⓒ Ⓓ Ⓔ	34 Ⓐ Ⓑ Ⓒ Ⓓ Ⓔ	49 Ⓐ Ⓑ Ⓒ Ⓓ Ⓔ	64 Ⓐ Ⓑ Ⓒ Ⓓ Ⓔ	79 Ⓐ Ⓑ Ⓒ Ⓓ Ⓔ
5 Ⓐ Ⓑ Ⓒ Ⓓ Ⓔ	20 Ⓐ Ⓑ Ⓒ Ⓓ Ⓔ	35 Ⓐ Ⓑ Ⓒ Ⓓ Ⓔ	50 Ⓐ Ⓑ Ⓒ Ⓓ Ⓔ	65 Ⓐ Ⓑ Ⓒ Ⓓ Ⓔ	80 Ⓐ Ⓑ Ⓒ Ⓓ Ⓔ
6 Ⓐ Ⓑ Ⓒ Ⓓ Ⓔ	21 Ⓐ Ⓑ Ⓒ Ⓓ Ⓔ	36 Ⓐ Ⓑ Ⓒ Ⓓ Ⓔ	51 Ⓐ Ⓑ Ⓒ Ⓓ Ⓔ	66 Ⓐ Ⓑ Ⓒ Ⓓ Ⓔ	81 Ⓐ Ⓑ Ⓒ Ⓓ Ⓔ
7 Ⓐ Ⓑ Ⓒ Ⓓ Ⓔ	22 Ⓐ Ⓑ Ⓒ Ⓓ Ⓔ	37 Ⓐ Ⓑ Ⓒ Ⓓ Ⓔ	52 Ⓐ Ⓑ Ⓒ Ⓓ Ⓔ	67 Ⓐ Ⓑ Ⓒ Ⓓ Ⓔ	82 Ⓐ Ⓑ Ⓒ Ⓓ Ⓔ
8 Ⓐ Ⓑ Ⓒ Ⓓ Ⓔ	23 Ⓐ Ⓑ Ⓒ Ⓓ Ⓔ	38 Ⓐ Ⓑ Ⓒ Ⓓ Ⓔ	53 Ⓐ Ⓑ Ⓒ Ⓓ Ⓔ	68 Ⓐ Ⓑ Ⓒ Ⓓ Ⓔ	83 Ⓐ Ⓑ Ⓒ Ⓓ Ⓔ
9 Ⓐ Ⓑ Ⓒ Ⓓ Ⓔ	24 Ⓐ Ⓑ Ⓒ Ⓓ Ⓔ	39 Ⓐ Ⓑ Ⓒ Ⓓ Ⓔ	54 Ⓐ Ⓑ Ⓒ Ⓓ Ⓔ	69 Ⓐ Ⓑ Ⓒ Ⓓ Ⓔ	84 Ⓐ Ⓑ Ⓒ Ⓓ Ⓔ
10 Ⓐ Ⓑ Ⓒ Ⓓ Ⓔ	25 Ⓐ Ⓑ Ⓒ Ⓓ Ⓔ	40 Ⓐ Ⓑ Ⓒ Ⓓ Ⓔ	55 Ⓐ Ⓑ Ⓒ Ⓓ Ⓔ	70 Ⓐ Ⓑ Ⓒ Ⓓ Ⓔ	85 Ⓐ Ⓑ Ⓒ Ⓓ Ⓔ
11 Ⓐ Ⓑ Ⓒ Ⓓ Ⓔ	26 Ⓐ Ⓑ Ⓒ Ⓓ Ⓔ	41 Ⓐ Ⓑ Ⓒ Ⓓ Ⓔ	56 Ⓐ Ⓑ Ⓒ Ⓓ Ⓔ	71 Ⓐ Ⓑ Ⓒ Ⓓ Ⓔ	86 Ⓐ Ⓑ Ⓒ Ⓓ Ⓔ
12 Ⓐ Ⓑ Ⓒ Ⓓ Ⓔ	27 Ⓐ Ⓑ Ⓒ Ⓓ Ⓔ	42 Ⓐ Ⓑ Ⓒ Ⓓ Ⓔ	57 Ⓐ Ⓑ Ⓒ Ⓓ Ⓔ	72 Ⓐ Ⓑ Ⓒ Ⓓ Ⓔ	87 Ⓐ Ⓑ Ⓒ Ⓓ Ⓔ
13 Ⓐ Ⓑ Ⓒ Ⓓ Ⓔ	28 Ⓐ Ⓑ Ⓒ Ⓓ Ⓔ	43 Ⓐ Ⓑ Ⓒ Ⓓ Ⓔ	58 Ⓐ Ⓑ Ⓒ Ⓓ Ⓔ	73 Ⓐ Ⓑ Ⓒ Ⓓ Ⓔ	88 Ⓐ Ⓑ Ⓒ Ⓓ Ⓔ
14 Ⓐ Ⓑ Ⓒ Ⓓ Ⓔ	29 Ⓐ Ⓑ Ⓒ Ⓓ Ⓔ	44 Ⓐ Ⓑ Ⓒ Ⓓ Ⓔ	59 Ⓐ Ⓑ Ⓒ Ⓓ Ⓔ	74 Ⓐ Ⓑ Ⓒ Ⓓ Ⓔ	89 Ⓐ Ⓑ Ⓒ Ⓓ Ⓔ
15 Ⓐ Ⓑ Ⓒ Ⓓ Ⓔ	30 Ⓐ Ⓑ Ⓒ Ⓓ Ⓔ	45 Ⓐ Ⓑ Ⓒ Ⓓ Ⓔ	60 Ⓐ Ⓑ Ⓒ Ⓓ Ⓔ	75 Ⓐ Ⓑ Ⓒ Ⓓ Ⓔ	90 Ⓐ Ⓑ Ⓒ Ⓓ Ⓔ

书面表达

请用黑色签字笔在答题区域内作答，超出黑色边框区域的答案无效！

样张（英语）

5

10

书 面 表 达　　　　　　请用黑色签字笔在答题区域内作答，超出黑色边框区域的答案无效！

15

20

25

30

LT-1/8R 2013B002B

Hi-Fi FATMD Test 5

PAPER ONE

Part I   Listening Comprehension (30%)

Section A

Directions: *In this section, you will hear fifteen short conversations between two speakers. At the end of each conversation, you will hear a question about what is said. The question will be read only once. After you hear the question, read the four possible answers marked A, B, C, and D. Choose the best answer and mark the letter of your choice on the* **ANSWER SHEET**.

Listen to the following example:

You will hear:

    W: I feel faint.

    M: No wonder. You haven't had a bite all day.

    Question: What's the matter with the woman?

You will read:

    A. She is sick.

    B. She was bitten by an ant.

    C. **She is hungry**.

    D. She spilled her paint.

    Here C is the right answer.

Sample Answer

A B ● D

Now let's begin with question Number 1.

1. A. John failed the exam.   B. John didn't take the exam.

    C. John passed the exam, but scored low.   D. It took John a long time to pass the exam.

2. A. To travel by train.   B. To go by taxi.

    C. To go hiking.   D. To rent a car.

3. A. 1-231-555-1212.   B. 1-213-555-2112.

    C. 1-213-555-1212.   D. 1-231-555-2112.

4. A. Morning sickness.   B. A frequent headache.

    C. A pain in her right leg.   D. A boring hospitalization.

5. A. Doctor and patient.   B. Boss and secretary.

    C. Agent and customer.   D. Driver and passenger.

6. A. To buy another pair of shoes.   B. To help his brother right away.

    C. To turn to his brother for help.   D. To seek advice from the woman.

7. A. He is offering a piece of advice.   B. He is examining a patient.

    C. He is attending his daughter.   D. He is taking a patient's history.

8. A. To ask the man to call her back.　　B. To go to the botanic garden.
   C. To do some gardening.　　D. To play tennis.

9. A. Louise is not a newcomer.　　B. Louise loves being a nurse.
   C. Louise did a lot of work for the man.　　D. Louise has been waiting for a long time.

10. A. Two.　　B. Three.
    C. Four.　　D. Seven.

11. A. She was thrown out of the car.　　B. She was knocked down by the car.
    C. She hit her head on the steering wheel.　　D. She got the steering wheel in her chest.

12. A. She overacted to the man.　　B. She cried over her failure.
    C. She made a success of diet.　　D. She was jealous of the man.

13. A. He hates those who fool around.　　B. He will never try the stuff.
    C. He will shoot any drug dealer.　　D. He regrets having tried the stuff.

14. A. The opposite to the man's expectation.　　B. A quicker recovery than expected.
    C. A pair of mismatching boots.　　D. Her healthy pregnancy.

15. A. He will do as requested.　　B. He will not join the team.
    C. The woman is crazy about him.　　D. The woman has trouble standing.

Section B

Directions: *In this part, you will hear three passages. After each one, you will hear five questions. After each question, read the four possible answers marked A, B, C, and D. Choose the best answer and mark the letter of your choice on the* **ANSWER SHEET**.

Sample Answer
A　B　●　D

Dialogue

16. A. For the purpose of diagnosis confirmation.　　B. For the possibility of legal trouble.
    C. For the doctor's investigation.　　D. For the patient's future use.

17. A. He has got cancer in his pancreas.　　B. He falls with a stomach problem.
    C. He suffers from fatigue.　　D. He has a loss of weight.

18. A. See a dietician.　　B. Have an operation.
    C. Start chemotherapy.　　D. Take medications for pain relief.

19. A. A couple of years.　　B. More than 5 years.
    C. A couple of months.　　D. Approximately 5 years.

20. A. Suspicious.　　B. Anxious.
    C. Hesitant.　　D. Factual.

Passage One

21. A. Life evolution.　　B. Space exploration.
    C. Extraterrestrial life.　　D. Unknown flying objects.

22. A. His 50th birthday.
    B. NASA's 50th anniversary.
    C. The University's 50th anniversary.
    D. The US Cosmology Association's 50th anniversary.

23. A. Even primitive life is impossible.　　B. Intelligent life is fairly common.
    C. Intelligent life is less likely.　　D. Any form of life is possible.

24. A. Nuclear weapons.　　B. Alien kidnapping.

C. Human extinction.

D. Dangerous infection.

25. A. Ironic.   B. Negative.

C. Indifferent.   D. Supportive.

Passage Two

26. A. Obese people need more food.   B. Obese people require more fuel.

C. Obesity contributes to global warming.   D. Obesity is growing as a global phenomenon.

27. A. Limited living space.

B. Crowded shopping malls.

C. Food shortages and higher energy prices.

D. Incidence of diabetes and cardiovascular diseases.

28. A. Over 700 millions.   B. Over 400 millions.

C. Over 2.3 billions.   D. Over 3 billions.

29. A. 1800 calories.   B. 1280 calories.

C. 1680 calories.   D. 2960 calories.

30. A. Climate change.   B. The fall of food prices.

C. A rise in energy prices.   D. An increasing demand for food.

Part Ⅱ Vocabulary (10%)

Section A

Directions: *In this section, all the statements are incomplete, beneath each of which are four words or phrases marked A, B, C, and D. Choose the word or phrase that can best complete the statement and mark the letter of your choice on the* **ANSWER SHEET**.

31. The _____ conditions and places are likely to cause diseases.

A. insanitary   B. insidious

C. insane   D. inefficacious

32. The witness was _____ by the judge for failing to answer the question.

A. abstained   B. acquitted

C. admonished   D. adduced

33. He has _____ two cars this year because of traffic accidents.

A. pulled off   B. worn out

C. passed out   D. written off

34. People are much better informed since the _____ of the Internet.

A. convenience   B. advent

C. interface   D. aftermath

35. All the instruments that came into contact with the patient must be _____ before being used by others.

A. sterilized   B. labelled

C. quarantined   D. retained

36. By adopting this cunning policy the clinic risks _____ many of its patients.

A. acquitting   B. allocating

C. alleviating   D. alienating

37. Humor can also be a powerful _____ against stress and misfortune.

A. bravery   B. blossom

C. buffer   D. buffet

38. Diabetes upsets the _____ of sugar, fat and protein.
    A. metastasis   B. metabolism
    C. malaise   D. maintenance

39. The muscular _____ can affect the way we feel mentally.
    A. potency   B. fiber
    C. lethargy   D. synthesis

40. Evidence is widespread that HIV-infected persons show reluctance to _____ their unsafe behaviours.
    A. respond to   B. reflect on
    C. wipe out   D. put off

Section B

Directions: *In this section, each of the following sentences has a word or phrase underlined, beneath which are four words or phrases. Choose the word or phrase which can best keep the meaning of the original sentence if it is substituted for the underlined part. Then mark your choice on the* **ANSWER SHEET.**

41. Memory can be both enhanced and impaired by the use of drugs.
    A. inhibited   B. injured
    C. induced   D. intervened

42. Is it true that this is the major drawback of the new medical plan?
    A. defect   B. assistance
    C. culprit   D. triumph

43. The physician was becoming exasperated with all the questions they were asking.
    A. frustrated   B. perplexed
    C. irritated   D. crippled

44. We were shocked at the physician's callous disregard for the human dimension of medicine.
    A. involuntary   B. apparent
    C. deliberate   D. indifferent

45. For years, biologists have known that chimpanzees and even some monkeys produce a panting sound akin to human laughter.
    A. rocking   B. gasping
    C. vibrating   D. resonating

46. Everybody at the party was in a very relaxed and jolly mood.
    A. rejoicing   B. reconciling
    C. refreshing   D. resenting

47. The bacterial infection is curable with judicious use of antibiotics.
    A. impudent   B. imprudent
    C. purulent   D. prudent

48. He tried to run, but he was hampered by his broken leg.
    A. endangered   B. endured
    C. encountered   D. encumbered

49. The whole holiday was a colossal waste of money.
    A. consecutive   B. conductive
    C. considerate   D. considerable

50. The idea of correcting defective genes is slightly not particularly <u>controversial</u> in the scientific community.

A. inevitable   B. applicable

C. disputable   D. incredible

Part III   Cloze (10%)

Directions: *In this section, there is a passage with ten numbered blanks. For each blank, there are four choices marked A, B, C, and D, listed on the right side. Choose the best answer and mark the letter of your choice on the* **ANSWER SHEET**.

Every day, over a million people log onto different Internet-based games. There is truly something for everyone in the gaming world. Games provide a quick escape from ___51___ . Game developers are the new breed of storytellers, creating alternative ___52___ . Games represent the ultimate interactive movie, allowing the user to control the direction of the plot.

And now the newest technologies allow you to play games no matter where you are. At home, we have PC or video game consoles. ___53___ , a desktop or laptop computer can be loaded with OS-bundled games or Web-based freebies. Even while travelling, there are many wireless computers, portable game devices, wireless phones and PDAs ___54___ .

Games are now pushing back all the ___55___ once placed upon them by technology, category, realism, location and time. These advances are helping to push games into the ___56___ of virtual reality. Thus, the stuff of science fiction novels is gradually emerging, the graphic aspects of the game quickly ___57___ . Initially, electronic games involved ___58___ moving blocks across a TV or computer screen. ___59___ the vast increases in processing power, games are quickly approaching three-dimensional realism. This power allows a developer to create a ___60___ world where a gamer can look around in full 360-degree vision.

51. A. society   B. reality
     C. dream   D. illusion

52. A. approaches   B. characters
     C. worlds.   D. mazes

53. A. In general   B. At present
     C. In reality   D. At work

54. A. to choose from   B. to choose
     C. choosing from   D. chosen

55. A. defects   B. drawbacks
     C. limitations   D. disadvantages

56. A. room   B. realm
     C. range   D. boundary

57. A. evolves   B. evolving
     C. evolved   D. evolve

58. A. simply   B. readily
     C. exceptionally   D. simultaneously

59. A. Aiding by   B. To aid by
     C. Aided by   D. To be aided by

60. A. human   B. original
     C. realistic   D. microscopic

Part IV   Reading Comprehension (30%)

Directions: *In this part there are six passages, each of which is followed by five questions. For each question there are four possible answers marked A, B, C, and D. Choose the best answer and mark the letter of your choice on the* **ANSWER SHEET**.

Passage One

Too much alcohol dulls your sense, but a study in Japan shows that moderate drinkers have a higher IQ than teetotalers.

Researchers at the National Institute for Longevity Sciences in Aichi Prefecture, 250 kilometers west of Tokyo, tested the IQs of 2000 people between the ages of 40 and 79. They found that on average, men who drank moderately—defined as less than 540 milliliters of sake or wine a day—had an IQ that was 3.3 points higher than men who did not drink at all. Women drinkers scored 2.5 points higher than female teetotalers.

The type of alcohol didn't influence the results. The volunteers tried a variety of tipples, which ranged from beer and whisky to wine and sake.

The researchers are quick to point out that the results do not necessarily show that the results do not necessarily show that drinking will make you more intelligent.

"It's very difficult to show a cause-effect relationship," says senior researcher Hiroshi Shimokata.

"We screened subjects for factors such as income and education, but there may be other factors such as lifestyle and nutritional intake."

Shimokata says that people who drink sakes, or Japanese rice wine, tend to eat more raw fish. This could be a factor in enhanced intelligence, as fish often contain essential fatty acids that have been linked to brain development. Similarly, wine drinkers eat a lot of cheese, which is not something Japanese people normally consume or buy. Shimokata says the high fat content of cheese is thought to be good for the brain.

If alcoholic drinks are directly influencing IQ, Shimokata believes chemicals such as polyphenols could be the critical factor. They are known to have antioxidant properties and other beneficial effects on ageing bodies, such as dilating constricted coronary arteries.

The study is part of a wider research project to find out why brain function deteriorates with age.

61. The Japanese study was carried out on _____.
    A. the development of IQ
    B. the secret of longevity
    C. the brain food in a glass
    D. the amount of healthy drinking
62. The Japanese researchers found a higher IQ in _____.
    A. female teetotalers than in male ones
    B. female drinkers than in male ones
    C. moderate drinkers
    D. teetotalers
63. When he says that it is very difficult to show a cause-effect relationship, Shimokata means that _____.
    A. the study failed to involve such variables as income and education
    B. he is doubtful of the findings of the investigation
    C. there are some other contributing factors
    D. the results were just misleading
64. From Shimokata's mention of fish and cheese we can infer that in enhancing intelligence _____.
    A. sake or wine is a perfect match for fish and cheese
    B. they promote the drinking effect of sake or wine
    C. they are not as effective as sake and wine
    D. sake or wine is not alone
65. Based on the study, Shimokata would say that _____.
    A. intelligence improves with age
    B. IQ can be enhanced in one way or another
    C. polyphenols in alcohol may boost the brain
    D. alcoholic drinks will make you more intelligent

Passage Two

Women do not avoid fighting because they are dainty or scared, but because they have a greater stake than men in staying alive to rear their offspring. Women compete with each other just as tenaciously as men, but with a stealth and subtlety that reduces their chances of being killed or injured, says Anne Campbell of the department of psychology at the University of Durham.

Across almost all cultures and nationalities, men have a much smaller role than women in rearing children."Males go for quantity of children rather than quality of care for offspring, which means that the parental investment of women is much greater," says Campbell. And unlike men, who can't be sure that their children have not been fathered on the sly by other men, women can always be certain that half an offspring's genes are theirs.

Women have therefore evolved a stronger impulse than men to see their children grow up into adults. Men's psychological approach is geared to fathering as many children as possible.

To make this strategy work and to attract partners, men need to establish and advertise their dominance over rival males. Throughout evolution this has translated into displays of male aggression, ranging in scale from playground fights to world wars.

Men can afford to take more risks because as parents they are more expendable. Women, meanwhile, can only ensure reproductive success by overseeing the development of their children, which means avoiding death.

"The scale of parental investment drives everything," says Campbell. "It is not that women are too scared to fight," she says. "It's more to do with the positive value of staying alive, and women have an awfully big stake not just in offspring themselves but in offspring they might have in the future," she says.

This means that if women do need to compete—perhaps for a partner—they choose low risk rules of engagement. They use indirect tactics, such as discrediting rivals by spreading malicious rumours. And unlike men who glory in feats of dominance, women do better by concealing their actions and their "victories".

But there is no doubt, says Campbell, that the universal domination of culture by males has exaggerated these differences in attitudes to physical aggression."The story we've always been told is that females are not aggressive," says Campbell. And when they are aggressive, women are told that their behaviour is "odd or abnormal".

66. For the sake of their children, according to Campbell, women _____.
    A. are reluctant to start wars
    B. cannot avoid being dainty or scared
    C. would rather get killed or injured in fighting
    D. do not fight with men under any circumstances
67. It can be learned from the passage that men and women _____.
    A. present different family values in the world
    B. show definite differences in parenting skills
    C. are genetically conditioned in educating their children
    D. take different psychological approaches to their children
68. Which of the following would men most probably be concerned about according to the passage?
    A. Life.   B. Parenting.
    C. Dominance.   D. Reproduction.
69. To avoid death, women _____.
    A. cannot afford to confront risks   B. choose to fight in a violent way
    C. try to seek protection from men   D. would resort to the "odd or abnormal" tactics
70. What is the main idea of the passage?
    A. Why men and women possess different parenting skills.
    B. Why men are more aggressive than women.

C. Why women evolve in their own way.

D. Why women do not start fights.

Passage Three

The first line reads: "She sits on the bed with a helpless expression. What is your name? Auguste. Last name? Auguste. What is your husband's name? Auguste, I think." The 32 pages of medical records that follow are the oldest medical description of Alzheimer's disease Psychiatrist Konrad Maurer and his colleagues at Johann Wolfgang Goethe University in Frankfurt found the file in their hospital's archive, where it had been missing for nearly 90 years, and published excerpts from it last May in *The Lancet*. The notes, in a cramped, archaic German script, were written by Alois Alzheimer—the physician who first described the disease.

His patient, Auguste D., was a 51-year-old woman who had suffered fits of paranoid jealousy and memory lapses so disturbing that her family finally brought her to a local hospital known as the Castle of the Insane. Over the next four years, Alzheimer tracked her condition. Upon her death he examined her brain tissue and found the distinctive lesions that are now hallmarks of the disease.

Today Alzheimer's afflicts some 4 million Americans. Although it still cannot be cured, or even treated very well, several recent studies hint that some treatments—from estrogen to vitamin E to anti-inflammatory drugs—can reduce either the risk of developing the disorder or its symptoms. And more is being learned about its distinctive pathology. This past year, for instance, researchers discovered a new kind of lesion in Alzheimer's patients. A genetic study also pinpointed a mutation that is present in some 60 percent of them—a mutation in the DNA of mitochondria, the energy-producing organelles of the cells.

But nearly a century ago, if it was Alois Alzheimer who first described the disease and in so doing became one of the first physicians to offer a biological basis for psychiatric condition. Finding the file, Maurer says, "is like holding history in your hands."

71. Obviously, the discovery of the missing file of Auguste D. _____.

    A. adds credit to Alois Alzhemier

    B. sheds doubt on the first description of Alzhemier's disease.

    C. presents a big challenge to the medical community

    D. has a great impact on the development of a cure for Alzhemier's disease.

72. The anatomical characteristics of Alzheimer's disease _____.

    A. can be found in the missing file

    B. could have been confirmed decades ago

    C. are wrongly described in the missing file

    D. even puzzle the medical community today

73. The findings of the research on Alzheimer's disease _____.

    A. sound encouraging   B. took more time than expected

    C. were ascribed to the missing file   D. will bring about a cure in no time

74. When he says that finding the file is like holding history in your hands, Maurer means _____.

    A. his assurance of the historical finding   B. his further studies on Alzheimer's disease

    C. the beauty of medical history   D. the importance of imagination

75. Which of the following can be the best title for the passage?

    A. The Physician Who First Described Alzheimer's disease.

    B. The Recent Studies on Alzheimer's disease.

    C. The Missing File of Auguste D..

    D. The History of Psychiatrics.

Passage Four

Dry-cleaning machines that use liquid carbon dioxide, as a solvent will go on sale in the US next year—thanks to chemists in North Carolina who have developed CO_2-soluble detergents. Dry-cleaners will lose their characteristic smell, and the new process will cut the amount of toxic waste produced in cleaning clothes.

Joseph DeSimone, a chemist at the University of North Carolina, Chapel Hill, says liquid CO_2 is an ideal solvent because after cleaning, the CO_2 can be evaporated off, collected, liquefied and reused.

The problem in developing the process, says DeSimone, has been that CO_2 by itself is not a good solvent. However, he points out that not much dissolves in water without the help of detergents, yet water is the most common solvent. What CO_2 needed, he thought, was the right detergent.

Detergent molecules such as those in washing-up liquid have two chemically distinct ends: one has a liking for water, the other sticks to dirt. Normal detergents do not dissolve in liquid CO_2, so DeSimone created three CO_2-soluble detergents. One end of the detergents has a fluorocarbon group, which makes them soluble in CO_2. The other end is soluble in water, oil or silicone, depending the type of the dirt being removed. The person doing the dry-cleaning has to decide which of the detergents is best suited for the job.

De-Simone's company, MiCell, will start selling liquid CO_2 dry-cleaning machines next year. They operate at room temperature at a pressure "about ten times the pressure of a bicycle tyre", according to a spokesman for MiCell.

Most dry-cleaners currently use chlorinated hydrocarbons such as perchloroethylene. But the US Environmental Protection Agency (EPA) is clamping down on the toxic waste emissions this produces. After cleaning with the new machines, the liquid CO_2 is evaporated and collected for reuse, leaving a residue of detergent and dirt.

Brad Lienhart, president of MiCell, says that cutting waste and pollution is the company's strongest selling point. "Dry-cleaner owners are saying 'get this burden off my back'," he says. He hopes to sell a hundred machines in the first year of business. About 15000 conventional dry-cleaning machines are sold around the world every year. Buster Bell, who owns Bell Laundry and Dry Cleaning in South Carolina, says the MiCell technology looks competitive, and he likes the reduced environmental impact. "You really don't know what is coming from the EPA," he says.

76. The passage begins with _____.
   A. a commercial advertisement　　　　　B. a horrible warning
   C. a sale promotion　　　　　　　　　　D. good news

77. What is the liquid CO_2 for?
   A. Better cleaning clothes.　　　　　　B. Helping recycle dry cleaners.
   C. Dissolving the toxic waste from dry cleaning.　　D. Reducing the toxic emission from dry cleaning.

78. The right detergent for CO_2 _____.
   A. makes dry cleaning easy　　　　　　B. must be chemically soluble
   C. is chemically of two purposes　　　　D. means a right person for dry-cleaning

79. When they are saying "get this burden off my back," the dry-cleaner owners refer to _____.
   A. the competition in the business of dry cleaning　　B. the pressure from EPA
   C. their potential profit　　　　　　　　D. their selling point

80. What is the strongest selling point of the MiCell technology according to Lienhart?
   A. It will promote dry-cleaning business.　　B. It is environment-friendly.
   C. It costs less in the market.　　　　　　D. All of the above.

Passage Five

The alarm on our household computer terminal rings and wakes me up. My husband simply stirs and goes back to sleep. I transfer today's information onto the personal data card I carry with me everywhere and scan today's readings. Values are given as to the number of litres of water I can use, the amount of coal-generated electricity I have been allocated and how many "envirocredits" I have earned.

I am free to use the water and electricity as I choose, however, I notice that the ration of electricity is decreasing every day. Of course, this will not be a problem when we have earned enough envirocredits to buy another solar panel. Envirocredits are earned by buying goods with limited or no packaging, minimizing the amount of garbage thrown out and by financially supporting "environtechnology". Before cars were phased out due to unpopularity, credits could be gained by using public transport.

I notice an extra passage added to the readings. At last I have been given permission to have a child almost instantaneously a package arrives with a label on it:"Anti-sterilization Unit". Inside there are instructions and a small device that looks like a cross between a pistol and a syringe. Eagerly I follow the instructions. The procedure is painless and I don't know if I am imagining it but I seem to feel the effects at once.

Shaking my husband awake, I tell him the good news. I want to get started baby-making right now."You've been on the waiting list for 37 years," he says, "Can't you wait until I've woken up properly?"

I decide that I probably don't have much choice and wander downstairs. I am feeling very privileged to have the opportunity to create a new life. It is saddening, however, when I realize that, because of strict population controls, this new life will be replacing an old one.

I decide to ring my mother and tell her the good news. When she answers the phone she is crying. She has received word that my grandmother has failed her latest health check and will die in a few days.

For some reason, I don't feel like creating that new life anymore.

81. Based on today's data, the wife will _____.
    A. use up all the envirocredits she earned
    B. make arrangements with her husband for the day
    C. be allowed to use a certain amount of water and electricity
    D. do as required to generate enough water and electricity for the day

82. According to the passage, envirocredits go to those who _____.
    A. recycle their garbage at home   B. limit themselves to solar energy
    C. push environtechnology forward   D. do something environment-friendly

83. The effects the wife is feeling at once following the instructions refer to _____.
    A. the desire to make a baby   B. the permission to make a baby
    C. the device to help her make a baby   D. the consequences of making a baby

84. The good news for the wife changes into bad news because _____.
    A. she has to wait for another 37 years   B. to create a new life is to replace an old one
    C. population is strictly controlled in the country   D. today she is not healthy enough to make a baby

85. What is the passage?
    A. It is a scenario.   B. It is a true story.
    C. It is a piece of news.   D. It is a scientific report.

Passage Six

Just because you're better educated doesn't mean that you're any more rational than everyone else, no matter how hard you may try to give that impression.

Take the selection of lottery numbers. A survey in Florida described at this year's annual meeting of the

American Association for the Advancement of Science shows that better educated people try to use random number systems to pick their lottery numbers.

Despite the apparent logic of choosing random numbers, however, their chances of winning are no better than those of ordinary folk who use birthdays, anniversaries and other "lucky" dates. Nor are they better off than those who draw on omens and intuitions, picking numbers seen on car number-plates and in dreams. But no doubt they feel a lot more rational.

That appearance of "rationality" may be a dangerous thing. Scientists are not immune to subtle and subjective influences on their judgments. Take the data from a survey of the public and members of the British Society of Toxicology discussed at the same meeting.

The survey showed that most people agree with the view that animals can be used to help predict how humans will react to chemicals, and that if a chemical causes cancer in an animal we can be "reasonably sure" it will cause cancer in humans. The toxicologists, however, are more circumspect. They accept the first statement but are less likely to agree that if a chemical causes cancer in an animal, it will do so in a human.

Can this difference be attributed to their expertise? Perhaps. But consider the considerable variation among toxicologists: those who were young, female, working in academia rather than industry or who felt that technology is not always used for the good of all, were more likely to agree that what causes cancer in an animal will cause cancer in a human.

Maybe we need to think more about how who we are affects our "rational" decisions.

86. According to the Florida-based survey, those who are better educated feel a lot more rational about the way they _____ .
   A. look at the world
   B. use logic in doing science
   C. choose their lottery numbers
   D. use numbers professionally and personally

87. Actually, the selection of random numbers _____ .
   A. does not work any better than the use of omens and intuitions
   B. stands more chance of winning a lottery in the United States
   C. is wrongly appreciated by rational people
   D. is widely practiced in lottery

88. What are the survey data suggesting in the passage?
   A. We are living in the age of rationality.
   B. Nobody can be trusted in terms of truth.
   C. Humans and animals do not react to chemicals in the same way.
   D. The sense of rationality cannot avoid being subjectively influenced.

89. What the author is trying to say in the passage _____ .
   A. can be further illustrated by the opinion among toxicologists
   B. is acceptable to those young and female toxicologists
   C. is rational enough to accept in the word of science
   D. has much to do with his own experience

90. Which of the following can be the best title for the passage?
   A. A Very Comforting Illusion.
   B. A Rational Approach to Lottery.
   C. A Survey on Education and Rationality.
   D. A Difference between Science and Others.

GO TO THE NEXT PAGE FOR PAPER TWO: WRITING.

PAPER TWO

Part V.　Writing (20%)

Directions: *In this part, there is an essay in Chinese. Read it carefully and then write a summary of 200 words in English on the* **ANSWER SHEET**. *Make sure that your summary covers the major points of the essay.*

答题要求

（1）紧扣主题，归纳总结；

（2）涵盖所有重要内容；

（3）避免选择原句进行简单翻译；

（4）无须推演或推论。

水果是可吃还是不可吃

　　水果含有人体必需而又不能自身合成的矿物质，具有强抗氧化作用、防止细胞衰老的维生素及可以明显降低血液中胆固醇浓度的可溶性纤维等，对人体健康十分有益。但中国人特别是男性，经常吃水果的比例很低。20 世纪 80 年代我在美国分析了美国 100 万人 10 年追踪研究的资料，发现不吃或很少吃水果的人群，肺癌病死率为吃水果人群的 1.75 倍。而且从 45 岁到 74 岁的每个 5 岁年龄组均出现类似的结果，说明这种因果关系非常可靠。美国有句谚语，"每天一苹果，医生远离我"，道出了水果对疾病的预防作用。世界卫生组织近年来提出了"天天五蔬果"的口号。其含义是，为保障健康，最好每天吃够五种蔬菜和水果。近年来美国哈佛大学的一些研究表明，多进食水果和蔬菜还可降低卒中和冠心病的发病危险。

　　那么，到底是水果中的什么成分起到了这样的作用？是不是维生素？服用市售维生素制剂是否可起到相同作用？我们又进一步分析了肺癌死亡与服用维生素制剂的关系。结果发现，经常服用维生素并不能起到类似的保护作用。再专门分析重度吸烟者肺癌病死率与进食水果和服用维生素制剂的关系，发现水果仍然起到保护作用，而维生素却没有。该分析研究的结论是人工合成的维生素不能替代水果对肺癌死亡的预防作用，后来的一些研究也得出了同样的结论。对此，营养免疫学专家的解释是：天然植物中的维生素并不是单独起作用，而是与其他维生素和营养素相互联合一起工作。一种维生素补充过多或不足，均会影响和削弱其他营养素或维生素的作用。由于化学合成的维生素是与其他维生素和营养素分离的，复方的各成分间的比例也与天然的不尽相同，所以它们不能产生与天然物质中所含的维生素一样的功效。有些国外的专家把这种现象戏称为"人造的不如自然造的"。另外，蔬菜水果中还可能含有某些尚未被人类认识的生理活性物质。目前，天然食物的抗氧化作用已成为一个重要的研究领域，各国营养学家正在进行研究开发。研究已证实，有些蔬菜水果具有强抗氧化作用，如大蒜、胡萝卜、柿子、柑橘、猕猴桃等能提高体内超氧化物歧化酶(SOD)的活性，发挥延缓衰老的作用。

　　综上所述，在日常生活中，水果应作为每日膳食的重要组成部分，绝不是可有可无的东西。对一般人群来说，维生素制剂绝不能也不应当代替日常对水果、蔬菜的进食。另外，过多地服用维生素制剂还可能引致一些副作用，有些甚至非常严重。如服用过量维生素 D 会导致软组织钙化，对肾脏和心血管系统造成损伤；长期服用维生素 E 易引致血栓等。在病态情况下，由于体内某些维生素的大量消耗或吸收合成转化不良，打破了其正常平衡，则必须适当补给。如发热、手术、患心肌梗死等疾病时需补充维生素 C；肝肾功能不良时需补充维生素 D 等。但这些均需在医生的指导下使用。

THIS IS THE END OF THIS OFFICIAL TEST.

Hi-Fi FATMD Test 5
Answer Keys
（非标准答案，仅供参考）

Part Ⅰ. Listening

1-3: DBC   4-6: CBC   7-9: BDA   10-12: BDA   13-15: BAB   16-18: DAB   19-21: CDC

22-24: BCD   25-27: DCC   28-30: ADB

Part Ⅱ. Vocabulary

31-35: ACDBA   36-40: DCDCB   41-45: BACDB   46-50: ADDDC

Part Ⅲ. Cloze

51-55: BBDAC   56-60: BBACC

Part Ⅳ. Reading

61-65: DCCDC   66-70: ADDAD   71-75: AAAAC   76-80: DCBBB   81-85: CDDBA

86-90: CADCB

Part Ⅴ. Writing

Is Fruit Indispensable or Replaceable?

It has been well-accepted that fruit is significant and indispensable to our health. However, with the rise of OTC synthetic vitamins, here comes the question of whether natural fruit is indispensable or replaceable. This essay is a brief discussion of the question.

Recently, WHO has advocated that people eat five kinds of vegetables and fruit every day because fruit contains many mineral substances, vitamins, soluble fibres that can prevent oxidation, aging of cells and reduce cholesterol in the bodies. Research shows that people eating little fruit die of lung cancer more than those who eat a lot of fruit by about 0.75 times.

However, what elements in fruit have such an effect a function? Is it vitamin? The answer is positive. But can OTC vitamins have similar function as fruit? Research finds that OTC vitamins fail to act as vitamins in fruit because the latter work together with other vitamins and nutrients in natural plants while the former act alone. That is why research reveals that OTC vitamins can replace fruit in reducing death rate of lung cancer. "Nature-made ones are better than man-made ones, " said some foreign experts. Besides, there are many bioactive substances in vegetables and fruit that are still unknown to man. Some fruit and vegetables such as oranges, garlic, pears, etc. can enhance the activity of SOD in the body and thus put off aging.

To conclude, fruit is an indispensable part of our daily diet and not replaceable by OTC vitamins. （247 words）

Tapescript for the Listening Comprehension

Section A

1.   M: Did you hear that John has passed Step One United States Medical Licensing Examination?

      W: Finally.

      Q: What does the woman imply?   D)

2. M: It's a one day trip. It must be pretty close!

    W: It's about four hours by train.

    M: Ha, OK. How else can we get there?

    W: I think the taxi only takes about two hours.

    M: I'm up for that.

    Q: What does the man prefer to do? B)

3. W: Information. What number do you need?

    M: I need the number of the German Embassy in Los Angeles.

    W: You have to dial information in Los Angeles. Dial 1-213-555-1212.

    M: Sorry. Could you say the number again?

    W: Sure, 1-213-555-1212.

    Q: What is the phone number? C)

4. W: Hello, Jim. I wonder if you could see a patient for me.

    M: Certainly, Anne. What's the story?

    W: Well, it's a Miss Linda Holmes, a thirty-five-year-old waitress. She is a frequent visitor. She came to see me this morning complaining a pain in her right leg.

    Q: What's the patient's complaint? C)

5. W: I'll be gone for a week. So I hope you can keep things straight around here.

    M: You have nothing to worry about.

    Q: What is the probable relationship between the two speakers? B)

6. W: If you see him as your brother, that's another pair of shoes. I suppose you can rely on him to help you.

    M: I know, but I feel ashamed to ask for his help.

    W: Don't think that way; he is your dear brother.

    M: Ok, I'll call him tonight.

    Q: What will the man probably do? C)

7. M: Would you like to get to the couch and lie on your back, please? Now I am going to take your left leg and see how far we can raise it. Keep the knee straight, does that hurt at all?

    W: Yes, just a little. Just slightly.

    Q: What is the man doing? B)

8. M: Hi Jane. This is Peter. It's such a nice day today! I thought we might go to the botanic garden（植物园）.

    W: I wish you had called me earlier. I've just made plans to play tennis.

    M: Oh, that's too bad. Maybe some other time.

    Q: What is the woman going to do? D)

9. W: How do you like the new nurse after the reception desk?

    M: You mean Louise? She has been here as long as I have.

    Q: What does the man imply? A)

10. M: Hello, Mrs. White. Is it your first visit to the clinic?

    W: Yes, but I've been to my doctor, and he's checked me over.

    M: I see from his letter that he is satisfied with the way things are going. Is this your first pregnancy?

    W: Oh, no. I've had three. I lost two and had two miscarriages.

    Q: How many children does the woman have now? B)

11. W: I've just been in a road accident.

    M: Were you thrown out of the car or did you get the steering wheel in your chest?

    W: I wasn't thrown out but I got the steering wheel in my chest, and I hit my head on the windscreen.

    M: Were you knocked out?

    W: I don't remember anything after the accident.

    Q: What can be said of the woman in the car accident?   D)

12. M: I am sorry to hear that you gained 20 pounds after going on a diet for two months.

    W: Don't cry crocodile tears. You would be jealous about my figure if I succeeded.

    Q: What can we say about the woman?   A)

13. W: Guess what? I hear some students at this school are fooling around with drugs.

    M: But you know, I'll stick to my guns and keep saying "no" to those who want me to try this stuff.

    Q: What does the man mean?   B)

14. M: How do you feel after the surgery? It seems that you've got a rebirth, right?

    W: I'm sorry, doctor. Honestly I think the shoe is on the other foot.

    Q: What does the woman mean?   A)

15. W: You have to stand up straight for 50 hours if you want to join this team.

    M: Are you crazy? What have I got myself into?

    Q: What does the man mean?   B)

Section B

Dialogue

    W: Mr. Scott, I like to record this consultation, so you and Mrs. Scott can play back later anything that may not be clear to you today. I'm afraid that the scan results aren't very good. It's likely that you've got a reoccurrence of cancer in your pancreas. That would explain why you've been feeling so tired and your loss of appetite and weight.

    M: Dr Smith, do I need surgery?

    W: Surgery isn't an option of this stage. Although we cannot operate, there are still a lot we can do to help you. You've got tablets for pain relief. And we can give you something stronger if you need it. We can also start you on a course of chemotherapy to help you with your symptoms. This won't cure you but will make you feel more comfortable. It's unusual to have any unpleasant side effects with this kind of chemotherapy. I'd like you to see a dietician for some advice on what you eat and to help you get your appetite back.

    M: What's my life expectancy? How long have I got?

    W: One can never be certain about these issues. People with this condition vary a great deal. I will be wrong to give you a definite time scale. But I'd say it's a matter of months rather than years. I'm sorry to have to tell you all this, but my feeling is it's always best to be honest with people and let you know what's what. If you're in an agreement, I'd like to book you into Ward 2 and start your chemo. You'll need to come in every week for the next month.

    16. What is the recorded consultation for?   D)

    17. According to the doctor's diagnosis, what has happened to Mr. Scott?   A)

    18. Which of the following is not a suggestion for Mr. Scott?   B)

    19. According to the doctor, what might be Mr. Scott's life expectancy?   C)

    20. Which of the following can best describe the tone of the doctor's words?   D)

Passage One

Steven Hawking: Life on other planets is likely, but intelligent life is less likely. Famed astrophysicist Stephen Hawking has been thinking a lot about the cosmic question, "Are we alone?" The answer is probably not, he says. If there is life elsewhere in the universe, Hawking asks why we haven't stumbled onto some alien broadcasts in space, maybe something like "alien quiz shows". Hawking's comments were part of the lecture at George Washington University on Monday in honor of NASA's 50th anniversary. He theorized that there are possible answers to whether there is extraterrestrial ET life. One option is that there likely isn't any life elsewhere. Or maybe there is intelligent life elsewhere, but it gets smart enough to send signals into space; it is also smart enough to make destructive nuclear weapons (核武器). Hawking said he prefers the third opinion: "Primitive life is very common and intelligent life is fairly rare," he then quickly added, "some would say it has yet to occur on earth."

So should you worry about aliens? Alien abduction claims come from "weirdos" and are unlikely. However, because alien life might not have DNA like us, Hawking warned: "Watch out if you meet an alien. You could be infected with a disease to which you have no resistance." The 66-year-old British cosmologist, who suffers from ALS and must speak through a mechanical device, believes "if the human race is to continue for another million years, we will have to boldly go where no one has gone before". Hawking compared people who don't want to spend money on human space exploration to those who opposed the journey of Christopher Columbus in 1492. "The discovery of the New World made a difference to the old. Just think we wouldn't have had a Big Mac or KFC."

21. What is the passage mainly about?   C)
22. What is the event when Hawking delivered his lecture at George Washington University?   B)
23. What is the idea Hawking favors in terms of extraterrestrial life?   C)
24. What is Hawking's warning to the encounter of an alien?   D)
25. What is Hawking's attitude towards human's space exploration?   D)

Passage Two

Obesity contributes to global warming, too. Obese and overweight people require more fuel to transport them and the food they eat. The problem will worsen as the population literally swells in size, a team at the London School of Hygiene & Tropical Medicine says. This adds to the food shortages and higher energy prices, the school's researchers wrote in the journal Lancet on Friday. At least 400 million adults worldwide are obese. The World Health Organization projects by 2015, 2.3 billion adults will be overweight and more than 700 million will be obese. In their model, the researchers pegged 40 percent of the global population as obese with a body mass index (BMI) of near 30. Many nations are fast approaching or have surpassed this level. BMI is a calculation of height to weight, and the normal range is usually considered to be 18 to/or 25, with more than 25 considered overweight and above 30 obese. The researchers found that obese people require 1,680 daily calories to sustain normal energy and another 1,280 calories to maintain daily activities, 18 percent more than someone with a stable BMI. Because thinner people eat less and are more likely to walk than to rely on cars, a slimmer population would lower demand for fuel for transportation and for agriculture. This is also very important because 20 percent of greenhouse gas emissions stem from agriculture. The next step is quantifying how much a heavier population is contributing to climate change, higher fuel prices and food shortages. "Promotion of a normal distribution of BMI would reduce the global demand for, and thus the price of food," Edward and Roberts wrote.

26. Which of the following can best describe the main idea of the talk?   C)

27. According to the talk, which of the following can be made worse by the growing obese population?　　C)

28. According to WHO, by 2015, what will be the estimated figure of the global obese population?　　A)

29. According to the researchers, how much energy does an obese person need for a day?　　D)

30. According to Edwards and Roberts, what would happen if we promote a normal distribution of BMI?　　B)

Part IV Wordlist for Clinical English

临床病历表格常用术语

1. 抗生素医嘱 Antibiotic Order

Prophylaxis	预防性用药
Duration of order	用药时间
Procedure	操作，手术
Empiric therapy	经验性治疗
Suspected site and organism	怀疑感染的部位和致病菌
Cultures ordered	做培养
Documented infection	明确感染
Site and organism	部位和致病菌
Explanation required	解释理由
Antibiotic allergies	何种抗生素过敏
No known allergy	无已知的过敏
Drug+dose+route+frequency	药名＋剂量＋途径＋次数

2. 住院/转院首页 Admission / transfer

Admit / transfer to	收入或转入
Resident	住院医师
Attending	主治医师
Condition	病情
Diagnosis	诊断
Diet	饮食
Activity	活动
Vital signs	生命体征
I / O	出入量
Allergies	过敏

3. 住院病历 Admission Case History

Identification	病人一般情况
Name	姓名
Sex	性别
Age	年龄
Marriage	婚姻
Person to notify and phone No.	联系人及电话

Race	民族
ID No.	身份证号码
Admission date	入院日期
Source of history	病史提供者
Reliability of history	可靠程度
Medical record No.	病历号
Business phone No.	工作单位电话
Home address and phone No.	家庭住地及电话
Chief complaint	主诉
History of present illness	现病史
Past Medical History	过往病史
Surgical	外科
Medical	内科
Medications	用药
Allergies	过敏史
Social History	社会史
Habits	个人习惯
Smoking	吸烟
Family History	家族史
Ob/Gyn History	婚姻/生育史
Alcohol use	喝酒
Review of Systems	系统回顾
General	概况
Eyes, Ears, Nose and Throat	五官
Pulmonary	呼吸
Cardiovascular	心血管
GI	消化
GU	生殖、泌尿系统
Musculoskeletal	肌肉骨骼
Neurology	神经系统
Endocrinology	内分泌系统
Lymphatic/Hematologic	淋巴系统/血液系统
Physical Exam	体检
Vital Signs	生命体征

P	脉搏
Bp	血压
R	呼吸
T	温度
Height	身高
Weight	体重
General	概况
HEENT	五官
Neck	颈部
Back/Chest	背部/胸部
Breast	乳房
Heart	心脏
Heart rate	心率
Heart rhythm	心律
Heart Border	心界
Murmur	杂音
Abdomen	腹部
Liver	肝
Spleen	脾
Rectal	直肠
Genitalia	生殖系统
Extremities	四肢
Cranial nerves	颅神经
Sensation	感觉
Motor	运动
Special P.E. on diseased organ system	专科情况
Radiographic Findings	放射
Laboratory Findings	化验
Lumbar puncture	腰穿
CT scan	CT扫描
MRI	核磁共振
Assessment	初步诊断与诊断依据
Summary	病史小结
Treatment Plan	治疗计划

4. 输血申请单 Blood Bank Requisition Form

(1) Reason for infusion	输血原因
▲红细胞	Packed red cells, washed RBCs
Hb<8.5	血色素<8.5
>20% Blood volume lost	>20%血容量丢失
Cardio-pulmonary bypass with anticipated Hb <8	心肺分流术伴预计血色素<8
Chemotherapy or surgery	血色素<10的化疗或手术者

with Hb <10	
Radiotherapy	放疗
▲全血	Whole blood
Massive on-going blood loss	大量出血
▲血小板	Platelets
Massive blood transfusion >10 units	输血10单位以上者
Platelet count <50×10³/μl with active bleeding or surgery	血小板<5万伴活动性出血或手术者
Cardio-pulmonary bypass with plt <100×10³/μl with active bleeding	心肺分流术伴血小板<10万，活动性出血者
Platelet count <20×10³/μl	血小板计数<2万
▲ Fresh frozen plasma	新鲜冰冻血浆
Documented abnormal PT or PTT with bleeding or Surgery	PT、PTT异常的出血或手术病人
Specific clotting factor deficiencies with bleeding/surgery	特殊凝血因子缺乏的出血/手术者
Blood transfusion >15units	输血>15个单位
Warfarin or antifibrinolytic therapy with bleeding	华法林或溶栓治疗后出血
DIC	血管内弥漫性凝血
Antithrombin III deficiency	凝血酶III缺乏
(2) 输血要求	Request for blood components
Patient blood group	血型
Has the patient had transfusion or pregnancy in the past 3 months?	近3个月，病人是否输过血或受孕过
Type and crossmatch	血型和血交叉
Units or ml	单位或毫升

5. 出院小结 Discharge Summary

Patient Name	病人姓名
Medical Record No.	病历号
Attending Physician	主治医生
Date of Admission	入院日期
Date of Discharge	出院日期
Principal Diagnosis	主要诊断
Secondary Diagnosis	次要诊断
Complications	并发症
Operation	手术名称
Reason for Admission	入院理由
Physical Findings	阳性体征
Lab/X-ray Findings	化验及放射报告
Hospital Course	住院诊治经过

Condition	出院状况	Incision type	切口类型
Disposition	出院去向	Healing course	愈合等级
Medications	出院用药	Operative (Non-operative)	手术（非手术）操作
Prognosis	预后	procedures	
Special Instruction to the	出院指导（饮食，活动量）	Nosocomial infection	院内感染
Patient (diet, physical activity)		Consultants	会诊医生
Follow-up Care	随访	Critical-No. of times	抢救次数
		Recovered-No. of times	成功次数

6. 住院 / 出院病历首页
Admission/discharge record

		Diagnosis qualitative analysis	诊断质量
Patient name	病人姓名	OP.adm. and discharge	门诊入院与出院诊断符合率
Race	种族	Dx concur	
Address	地址	Clinical and pathological	临床与病理诊断符合率
Religion	宗教	Dx concur	
Medical service	科别	Pre- and post-operative	术前术后诊断符合率
Admit (discharge) date	入院（出院）日期	Dx concur	
Length of stay	住院天数	Dx determined with in 24	入院后 24 小时（3 天）内
Guarantor name	担保人姓名	hours (3 days) after admission	确诊
Next of kin or person to notify	需通知的亲属姓名	Discharge status	出院状况
Relation to patient	与病人关系	Recovered	治愈
Previous admit date	上次住院日期	Improved	好转
Admitting physician	入院医生	Not improved	未愈
Attending physician	主治医生	Died	死亡
Admitting diagnosis	入院诊断	Disposition	去向
Final (principal) diagnosis	最终（主要）诊断	Home	家
Secondary diagnosis	次要诊断	Against medical ad	自动出院
Adverse reactions	副作用（并发症）	Autopsy	尸检
(complications)		Biopsy	活检
		Transferred to	转院到

Part V Wordlist for Listening Test(2024 新版)

常用听力词汇表

1. 各类英语考试听力部分易混、易错词汇表

address	发表演说；向…讲话；地址
advisor	(学生的)顾问，辅导员
agreeable	宜人的，令人愉快的
alarm	闹钟 (alarm clock)
album	唱片集；相册；邮册
announce	告知；公布
anxious	忧虑，紧张；不安；渴望
assistantship	助教奖学金
attractive	有魅力的，美丽的
balcony	楼座(很差的座位，与 orche-stra section 对应)阳台
beat	胜过，超过；难倒，使困惑
benefit	津贴；义演，慈善演出
box office	票房
broke、penniless	身无分文
cafeteria	学生食堂
can	罐
carry	(商店)出售，有货
cassette	磁带，盒式磁带
catalog	课程介绍；表格；清单
catching	有感染力的
claim check	(领取物品)存根、凭证
clear	天晴
coed	男女同校的；男女同住的宿舍楼
commons	厅，楼厅
confront	便面临令人不快的事；搭配
convention	年会
correspondence	信函
course	课程；高尔夫球场；时间段
court	球场
credits	学会；信任
deliver	送(货)

deserted	无人的；门庭冷落的
develop	冲洗(胶卷)
dietitian	(学生食堂的人)师傅
dominate	控制，占上风
doubt	不认为
down	细小而柔软
dressing	调味品
driveway	家门前
drugstore	杂货铺
due	到期，预期的；
dues	会费
elective	选修课
enrollment	学生人数
establish	使人们接受
exercise	体育锻炼，健身
expect	预料，认为
extension	推迟交作业的时间
fan	迷；扇子
fare	交通费
fascinating	极有趣的
film	胶卷(电影一般用 movie)
finals	期末考试
fire	解雇,(常见的同义词: lay off, let go, boot out, release, remove 等)
fitness	身体健康情况 (fitness center 健身中心)
fix	修理,准备,确定,弄来
forward	寄送
frontier	边远山区
frosting	(糕点上的)糖霜
garage	国库,修车厂
grade	分数,成绩,改(卷),打分
helping	一份食物
hire	雇佣
hurt	疼痛

issue	一期（刊物）；（有争议的）问题；发行（布）	record	唱片
job offer	打工机会	reference	推荐人
light	清淡的，易消化的；有光亮的；轻的	requirement	必修课
line	购物排成队	reserve book	保留书（指十分常用的书，借阅时间一般为 2～24 小时，否则罚款）
load	负荷，负载；选修课	return	回球
locate	找到	ride	搭车
locker	（浴室、健身房内等）有锁的小柜	save	占位子；预留，保留
		savings account	储蓄账号
look	表情，神色	season	赛季
lot	地皮	serve	发球
measure	取一定数量的东西	shame	遗憾，可惜，失望
meet	（接人），见面；上课	silverware	餐具
model	型号；款式	sketch	素描，速写
nerve	胆量，勇气	skip	略过，漏过，遗漏
newsstand	报（书）摊	solid	纯的，色彩一样的；稳定（固）的
orchestra section	（剧院中）最好的座位		
off	离开，不…	sort	分类，归类
orientation	新生熟悉环境	spell	一段时间；身体不适的时间
outgoing	开朗的，外向的，好交际的；友好的	spot	看到，认出
		spotless	非常干净，一尘不染
paper	论文；报纸；(papers 档案材料)	spread	床罩，罩布等
pass	票证；放弃，不要	stack	书库；堆、垛
performance	表现；表演	stamp	盖章
pocketbook	（女士用）包；钱包	standstill	停顿，停止
policy	保险单	straw	吸管
polish	鞋油，上光剂；擦亮，修饰	supplies	生活必需品；用品
poster	装饰画；海报	suspect	认为（肯定的语气）
pour	下大雨	tape	透明胶，胶带纸
prerequisite	基础课	teller/cashier	出纳，收银员
presentation	发言，讲话，演说（会议和上课）	terrific	极好的
program	节目单	ticket	交通罚款单
project	课题项目，作业	tie	平局（比赛）；领带
promise	光明的前途	trace	少许，微量
punch	混合甜饮料；打孔，剪票	track	足迹，痕迹；追踪，探索
pushover	容易对付的人；容易被利用的人	trail	山间小道
		tray	学生自助食堂的托盘
quarter	三个月；25 美分；季刊	treasurer	生活部长（学生会）
race	比赛；快速移动	treat	招待，请客；付钱；治病，治疗
raise	集资，积聚；涨工资		
rate	规定的费用和价格；比率，利率	upset	打翻；感到心烦
		utilities	水电费；用具
rating	收视率或受欢迎程度	vacuum	吸尘
recall	回忆，回想起；收回	view	视野，观看；风景
receiver	电话听筒	want ad	广告
reception	招待会	wing	配楼
receptionist	接待人员（小姐）	workshop	互相交流的课程
recommend	推荐，推崇；喜欢	yearbook	毕业纪念册，毕业留言簿

2. 听力部分常见词组

A

a busy signal	（电话）忙音
a close call	侥幸地脱险
a far cry from	很大的差异
a fish out of water	处在陌生环境中的人，不知其所的人
a narrow escape	九死一生，死里逃生
a piece of cake	容易的事
a stone's throw	一箭之遥，短距离
a while back	几个星期或几个月以前；不久以前
abide by	遵守；坚持
abound in (with)	有大量的；富于；充满
above all	首先；尤其
above (over) the heads of	深奥得使（听众等）不能理解
absence of mind	心不在焉
absent oneself from	缺席，未参加
according to	按照；根据…所说
account for	说明（原因等）；解释
acquaint oneself with (of)	知道，熟悉于…的对面
across from	在…的对面
act as	充当；扮演…的角色，起…的作用
act for	代理；代办
add fuel to the fire (flame)	火上加油
ass up	加起来，合计
adhere to	坚持；遵守
adjust oneself to	使自己适应于
after all	毕竟，终究，终归
after hours	工作（学习）完毕后，下班以后
after one's (own) heart	正合自己的心意
after while	等一会儿；不久
again and again	再三地，反复地
against one's will	违背意愿地，违心地
against sb's grain	（跟某人的性格、感情或愿望）格格不入
agree with	与…相符合；同意
ahead of schedule	提前
ahead of time	在原定时间以前，提前
alarm system	警报系统
all along	始终，一直
all at once	突然
(all) at sea	茫然，不知所措
all day (long)	一天到晚，整天地

all in all	总的说来
all in a day's work	常事；习以为常
all night (long)	整夜
all of a sudden	突然，出乎意料地
all one's life	一生，终身
all over oneself	非常高兴，非常满意
all the more	更加，益发
all the same	（虽然…）还是，仍然
all the time	一直，始终
all the year round	一年到头，终年
all there	头脑清醒的（常用于否定句）
all too well	非常好
all wet	完全搞错了，大错特错
along with	与…一道，和
and all that	诸如此类
and how	当然，那还用说
another pair of shoes	另外一回事
anything but	根本不…，决不…
apart from	除…以外
apply for	申请
approve of	赞同，认可
apt at	善于，长于
apt to	易于，有…的倾向
argue sb. into (doing) sth.	说服某人做某事
argue sb. out of (doing) sth.	说服某人不做某事
around the clock	昼夜的，连续二十四小时的
as a rule	通常；一般说来
as a matter of fact	事实上，其实
as a whole	整个来说，总体上
as cool as cucumber	十分镇静
as far as	就…来说，至于
as fit as a fiddle	非常健康，精神焕发
as luck would have it	碰运气，碰巧
as soon as	一…就…
as usual	像往常一样，照例
ask out	邀请外出吃饭
associate with	与…交往；和…联系在一起
at a discount	低于正常价格；打折扣
at (in) a distance	在远处
at a loss	困惑，不知所措；亏本地
at a time	每次，一次
at any (all) cost	不惜任何代价；无论如何
at (one's) ease	自由自在地，不受拘束；不紧张
at home	自在，不拘束
at last	终于，最后
at no time	在任何时候都不，从不，决不
at odds	争吵，不和；不一致

at once	同时，马上，立刻	be free to	可随意做
at one's wit's end	智穷计尽；不知所措	be good at	擅长
at present	现在，目前	be hard up	穷，缺钱
at random	随便地，任意地	be hard on (upon)	对…严厉（苛刻）的
at risk	在危险中	be in harmony with	符合，一致
at sb's disposal	由某人做主；供某人使用	be in charge (of)	主持，负责
at sb's service	听候某人吩咐；听凭某人	be in fashion	流行
	使用	be in force	生效
at short notice	一得到通知（就马上…）	be in sb's shoes	处于某个的地位（境遇）
at sixes and sevens	乱七八糟；意见不一致	be in season	（蔬菜水果等）当令；上市
at stake	在危险中；处于成败（存亡，	be known to	为…所熟知
	输赢）关头	be likely to	可能
at table	在进餐	be meant for sb	命中注定
at (the) least	至少，最低限度	be prepared for	准备好，做…打算
at the mercy of	完全受…支配，任凭…摆布	be relevant to	和…有关联
at the moment	此刻（用于现在时中）；那时	be sensitive to	对…敏感
	（用于过去时中）	be sick of	讨厌
at (the) most	至多，不超过	be subject to	易受…影响；视…而定
at the risk of	冒着…危险	be suitable for	适合于
at the same time	同时；一齐	be the worse for	变得更坏；因…而更坏
at (the) sight of	一看见	be true to	忠于，信守；与…丝毫不差
at (on) the tip of one's tongue	差一点说出；几乎想起	be under the impression	以为
at times	有时，偶尔；不时	be up	起身，离床；不睡觉
attend to	照料；安排，处理	be up to	胜任；忙于
attribute to	把…归因于；是…的结果	be up to one's neck in work	工作太多，忙不过来
auditing course	旁听课程	be up to sb	由某人决定
avail oneself of	利用，趁（机会）	be well-known to	众所周知
a while back	不久以前	be wrong with	有问题，有毛病
		bear with	宽容，耐心等待

B

		beat around (about) the bush	拐弯抹角地说或做；旁敲侧击
		because of	因为，由于
back out (of)	退出；收回（诺言等）；倒车	before long	不久；很快
back up	支持，援助；阻塞	behind the times	过时的；落伍的
be absorbed in	全神贯注于，专心于	believe in	信任，信赖
be all ears	全神贯注地倾听着	belong to	属于；为…之财产
be all set	准备就绪；已下决心	benefit concert	义演音乐会
be all the same	完全一样，毫无区别	beside oneself	失常，忘形，发狂
be all thumbs	笨拙的，笨手笨脚的	best of all	最，首先，第一
be all aware of	知道，觉察到；意识到	bet on the wrong horse	估计（判断）错误
be beside oneself with joy	得意忘形	better off	更富有；境况更好
be booked up	客满，没有空位；没有时间	between ourselves	只限于咱俩之间（别对外
be busy doing sth.	正忙于做（某事）	(you and me)	人讲）
be cross with	生气，不高兴	beyond belief	难以置信地；超出想象地
be engaged in	忙于，致力于	beyond compare	无可比拟；无双
be enthusiastic about	热心于	beyond control	无法控制，难以控制
be fed up with	吃得过饱，感到腻味（厌烦）	big shot	大人物，大亨，要人
be fond of	喜欢，爱好	bird in the hand	已到手的东西；有把握的事物
be free of	免除，脱离	bit by bit	逐渐地，一点一点地
		bite off more than one	去做自己做不了的事；自不

can chew	量力	by leaps and bounds	飞跃地,极迅速地
blow one's top	生气,气愤	by (on) lease	以租赁方式
blow up	发脾气,暴怒;放大(照片等)	by mistake	弄错,失误
		by night	在夜间;趁黑夜
blue in the face	恼怒	by no means	决不,一点也不
boil down to	归根结底	by now	此刻(已经);现在
book up	订(座、票);预定(房间等)	by oneself	独自地;独力地,全靠自己地
bound for	准备到…去的;(船等)开往…的	by reason of	由于,因为,凭…的理由
branch out	扩充范围;扩大规模;向新的方向发展	by sea	由海路;乘船
		by the sea	在海边,在海崖上
brand new	全新的	by the way	顺便提一下;另外
bread and butter	生活来源,生计	by turns	轮流;交替地
break a (the) record	打破纪录;打破前例	by way of	经由;用…方式
break down	中止,停顿;发生故障		

C

break fresh (new) ground	开辟新天地;打破惯例
break in	闯入;使(新物体)逐渐合用;插嘴
break off	暂停工作,休息
break one's word	失信,食言;毁约
break out	突然发生;爆发
break sb's heart	使某人伤心(悲痛、绝望)
break the ice	打破沉默;打开僵持的局面
break up	分解;解散;关系断绝
bring about	带来,引起
bring around (round)	使恢复知觉(健康)
bring forward	提出(问题、建议等)
bring into force	使开始生效,开始实行
bring to an end	结束,终止(某事)
bring to light	揭示;发现,发掘
bring up	抚养;培养;使成长
brush up on	温习;重新练习
build up	逐步建立,树立;集结;增大
bump into	偶然碰上,不期而遇
burn a hole in sb's pocket	(钱)在某人口袋里留不住
burn oneself out	筋疲力尽
burn out	把…烧坏;把…烧光
burn the midnight oil	学习(工作)到深夜;开夜车
burn up	发怒,激怒;(使)烦躁
by accident	偶然;意外地,无意中
by air	坐(乘)飞机
by all means	当然,一定,毫无疑问地
by and by	不久以后,不一会儿
by chance	偶然,意外地,碰巧
by day	在白天,日间
by degrees	逐渐地;一步一步地
by fits and starts	一阵一阵地;不规则地
by half	非常,相当
by heart	凭记忆;熟记
by land	由陆路

call a spade a spade	直言不讳
call after	以…命名
call at	拜访(某家、某地)
call back	回电话
call for	要求,需要
call it a day	收工,休息,终止
call it a night	下工;回家
call off	取消
call on	访问、拜访(某人)
call the roll	点名;按名册点名
call up	打电话
calm down	(使)平静下来;(使)镇定下来
can do with	将就;能对付;满足于
can not but	不得不
can not help (doing)	不能不;禁不住
can not help oneself	不能抑制自己
capable of	有…能力的;能…的
card catalog	卡片目录
care for	喜欢
carry away	拿走;迷住
carry coals to Newcastle	多此一举;白费力气
carry out	贯彻,执行
carry the house	博得全场喝彩
carry through	进行(到底),完成;使渡过难关
carry too far	做得过分,走极端
cash in on	利用时机获利;生财有道
cast away	丢掉,抛弃
cast down	扔掉,抛下;使沮丧
catch (a) cold	伤风,感冒
catch a glimpse of	瞥见
catch (a) sight of	看到,忽然看见

catch fire	着火，烧着；突然流行起来	consist in	在于，存在于
catch hold of	抓住；占有	consist of	由…组成，由…构成
catch on	变得流行；受欢迎	consult with	与…商量
catch on to	理解，明白	count in	算上某人，包括
catch one's breath	喘口气；放松一下	count on (upon)	依靠；期望，指望
catch one's eye	引人注目	count out	把…不计在内；把（某人）作
catch up on	赶做（尚未做的或忘了做		不参加论
	的事）	count up	把…加起来；共计
catch up with	急起直追；赶上	cram for	赶功课；临时准备应考
change one's mind	改变主意（或计划）	cross a bridge before	事未临头先发愁，杞人忧天
check in	办理登记手续；签到，报到	(until) one comes to it	（常用于否定句）
check out	付账后离开（旅馆等）；办理	cross one's mind	（念头等）出现于脑中；想起
	登记手续借出（书等）	cross out	划掉，删去；取消
cheer up	（使）高兴，（使）愉快；（使）	cry over spilt milk	作无益的后悔
	振奋）	cut corners	节省；走捷径
choral group	合唱团	cut down	削减；删节；删减
clean out	把…打扫干净；把…扫而光	cut it out	结束，停止（争吵等）；住口
clean up	把…收拾（打扫）干净	cut off	通电话时线路被切断；中断
clear off	清除，清理	cut off a corner	抄近路
clear up	整理，收拾，打扫；（天气）	cut out	剪掉；删掉
	变晴	cut short	突然停止；突然结束
close down	（工厂、企业等）关闭，停业，	cut to the bone	大大削减（价格、费用等）
	歇业		
cold shoulder	冷遇；冷淡对待		

D

come about	发生，出现	daily round	日常事务，日常例行工作
come across	偶然碰见；无意中发现	day after day	日复一日地，天天
come along	进展，进步	day and night	日日夜夜，夜以继日地
come around (round)	改变主意；接受别人的看法	day in and day out	每天；始终；经常
come down with	患…病，病例	day off	休息日，歇工（休假）的日子
come into	获得；继承（财产等）	dead beat	精疲力竭的
come into action	开始行动，开始运转	dead easy	很容易
come into contact (with)	和…联系；触及	dead tired	非常疲倦
come into fashion	流行起来	deal in	经营，做…买卖
come on	开始，出现，来临	deal with	论述，关于；与…交易
come straight to the point	开门见山（说话不转弯抹角）	decide against	决定不做…；判决…败诉
come through	获得成功	decide for	决定做；判决…胜诉
come to a head	（时机、事情等）成熟；迫近	depend on (upon)	依靠，依赖；取决于
	严重的关头	deprive of	使失去，剥夺，夺去
come to an end	结束，终止	despite of	不管，尽管
come to light	发现，真相大白	devote oneself to	献身于；专心致力于
come to nothing	失败，落空，终成泡影	die away	逐渐消逝（减弱，停止）
come to terms	达成协议；让步，妥协	die down	渐渐消失（减弱，熄灭，平息）
come to the point	说到要点，谈到问题的实质	die of	死于（疾病，饥饿，寒冷，虐
come true	实现；梦想成真		待等）
come up to	达到；符合；比得上	die out	消失，不复存在；灭绝
come up with	建议；提出	differ from	与…不同
come what may	不管发生什么事，无论如何	dig up	（经调查研究或费力地）发
compare notes	商量；交换意见		现，查出，得到
comply with	遵守，服从		
concentrate on	集中精力于		

dirt cheap	极便宜地	drop by (in)	非正式访问,顺便来访
dispose of	抛掉,除掉,处理掉	drop off	(让…)下车
do away with	废除;去掉;摆脱	drop out	退学;放弃;离去
do business with	和…做生意;和…交往	drop straight	结果很好,终于好转,恢复
do in a pinch	凑合用一下		正常
do in Rome as Rome does	入乡随俗	due to	由于,因为
do justice to	公正地对待;处理适当	dust out	急退
do one's best	竭尽所能;尽力	Dutch auction	拍卖者自动落价,直到发现
do one's bit	尽自己本分;尽自己的一份		有人愿意出资购买的拍卖
	力量	duty bound	理当去做;理应如此
do one's duty	尽职;尽本分;尽义务	dwell in the memory	记忆犹新
do over	重做	dwell on (upon)	详论,详述
do right	做得对		

E

do sb. a favour	帮某人的忙	each and every	每一个(加强语气用)
do sb. good	对某个有好处	each other	相互,彼此
do sb. harm	对某个有坏处	early bird	早起的人;早到者
do sth .a thousand times	某事反复使人生厌或不忘记	early on	早些时候,前不久;在初期
do the trick	达到预期目的;获得成功;	early or late	迟到
	发生效力	ease off	减轻,缓和(痛苦、负担、紧
do the honors	荣誉主持		张状态等)
do time	坐牢	ease up	减轻,放松;(风雨等)缓和
Don't cross that bridge	别杞人忧天	eat away	痛快地吃;继续吃下去;侵
until you come to it			蚀;蚕食
do up	包扎;捆好,束起	eat into	(酸、锈等)把…腐蚀掉;耗
do (go) without	无需;没有…也行,勉强对		费(钱财等)
	付过去	eat one's fill	饱食,尽量吃
do wrong	做错事;做坏事	eat (swallow) one's words	收回前言,承认说错
Do you think it'll help?	你觉得这样做有用吗?	eat out	在外吃饭;侵蚀;吃光
double duty	两种用途;双重目的(任务)	eat up	把…吃光;用尽,消费掉
down in the dumps (mouth)	沮丧的,忧郁的,心灰意	egg (edge) sb.on	怂恿,挑唆(某人做某事)
	懒的	elective courses	选修课程
down to earth	实事求是的;合理的	eligible for	合格,有资格
doze off	打瞌睡,打盹儿	end for end	反过来,掉个头
drag on (out)	(使)拖长;拖延	end in	以…为结果,以…结束,
drag one's feet (heels)	故意拖延;进展缓慢		终归
drama club	戏剧俱乐部	end in talk	终于成为空谈
draw a (the) line	区别、限制	end to end	头尾相接地,互相衔接地
draw a red herring across	转移讨论中心;分散谈话中的	end up	结束,结尾;终于(成为)
the track	注意力	engage in	参加,从事
draw lots	抽签	engage (oneself) to	和…订婚(常用于被动语态)
draw near	接近,临近	enjoy oneself	过得快乐
draw on	支取,动用;接近,临近	enter (one's name,	(报名)参加…竞赛;加入
draw (attract) sb's attention	引起某人的注意	oneself) for	
dress up	穿上盛装;乔装打扮	entitle sb. to	使某人有…有资格(或
drink like a fish	豪饮,牛饮		权力)
drive at	意指,意欲		
drive sb. mad (crazy)	使某人发疯		
drive sb. up the wall	大伤脑筋;使发狂;使烦恼		
drop a hint	暗示		
drop a line	写(短)信	escape one's lips	(话)溜出某人之口

estimate at	估计（数目、价钱、大小等）为…	fall sick (ill)	生病
even chance	胜败各半，成败相等	fall through	失败；毁灭
even if (though)	即使纵然，即使如此	fall to	开始，着手
even so	虽然如此，即便如此	fall to pieces	粉碎；崩溃
even up	（使）平衡；（使）拉平（相等）	fall under	被列为，归入…一类
ever after	自…以后，以后一直	familiar to	为…所熟悉
ever since	从那时起，自那时以来	familiar with	熟悉，通晓
every once in a while	时常，常常	familiarize oneself with	使自己熟悉（通晓）
every other	每隔一；隔一个地	far and wide	到处，四面八方
every so often	时常，不时	far cry	不大相同的东西；很大的差异
every time	每次，总是	far from	远离；远远不；完全不
except for	除…外；若无	far from it	远非如此，绝不是那样，一点也不
exclusive of	除…外，不把…计算在内		
excuse oneself	替自己辩解；请求原谅；请求允许离开	feed back	反馈；（听众等）反响，反应
excuse sb. from	同意某人不…，使某人免除（责任、惩罚等）	feed on (upon)	用…喂养；靠吃…过活
		feel cheap	觉得身体不舒服；感到羞愧
expand one's horizons	开阔眼界	feel like	很想要，恨不得
explain oneself	说明自己的意思；解释清楚	feel like a million (dollars)	健康和精神处于极好状态
express mail	快递	feel one's way	摸索着走；谨慎行事
express oneself	表示自己的意见；表达自己的意思	feel run-down	觉得筋疲力尽
		feel strange	觉得不舒服；觉得不习惯
		feel up to	觉得能胜任（常用于否定句或条件句）

F

		few and far between	稀少，罕见
		fight one's way	打开一条出路；奋斗前进
		figure out	算出；领会到，理解
face the music	承担后果；受到惩罚	fill in	填写；填满
face to face	（和…）面对面；当面	fill in for	暂时代替，补缺
face up to	勇于对付；大胆地面对	fill out	填写（表格）
fair and square	公正的，正大光明的	fill sb. in on	对某人提供关于…的事实（详情）
fair-weather friend	只能共安乐不能共患难的朋友		
fall apart	崩溃，瓦解；破裂	fill the bill	完全符合要求，解决问题
fall asleep	入睡，睡着	fill the prescription	给药方配药
fall back on (upon)	求助于，转而依靠	fill up	加满（油等）
fall behind	落后，跟不上；拖欠 (with)	financial aid (assistance)	经济资助
fall (sit) between two stools	失掉机会，两头落空	find fault with	挑剔；抱怨
fall down	跌倒；倒塌	find out	找出，发现
fall flat	不能引起兴趣；完全失败	finish up	结束，完成
fall for	听信；迷恋	finish up with	以…结束
fall in	掉进，跌入；（债务等）到期；（租约等）满期	fire escape	太平梯
		first and foremost	首先，首要
fall in love (with)	爱上，喜爱	first class	第一类邮件（或密封邮件）
fall in with	赞同；与…一致	first of all	第一，首先
fall into a decline	衰退，衰弱	first thing	作为第一件要做的事；首先
fall into the (a) habit of	养成…习惯	fit in with	（使）适合，（使）符合，（使适应）
fall (go down) on one's knees	跪下，屈膝		
fall on a sleep	麻木	fit the bill	满足（符合）要求，适合需要
fall short (of)	缺乏，不足；不符合	flatter oneself	自以为，自吹
		flesh and blood	血肉之躯；人类

flick (flip) through	将（书等）一翻而过，浏览	from (the) beginning to (the) end	自始至终，从头到尾
flip out	失去理智，发疯，发狂	from (the bottom of) one's heart	衷心地，真诚地
fly by	飞逝	from time to time	时常；不时，偶尔
fly off the handle	勃然大怒	full of go	劲头十足，精力旺盛
focus on	对焦点；集中在	full of years	老了，上了年纪
fold one's arms	袖手旁观，置身事外		
follow after	追求；力求达到		
follow one's nose	一直向前走，笔直走		
follow sth. through to completion	善始善终		

G

follow suit	照样做，仿效	gain (have, get) an advantage over	占优势
follow the fashion	赶时髦，迎合时尚	gain (get, have) the upper hand (of)	控制，掌握，占…上风
fool about (around)	闲荡，无所事事		
for a change	为了改变一下；为了换换花样	gain time	（钟表等）走得快
for a time	暂时；一度	gain weight	增加体重
for a while	暂时，一会儿	gammer (away) at	（不断）致力于，埋头于
for ages	很久，好久	get a line on	得到关于…的消息（知识、情况）；打听明白（某个或某事）
for all I care	与我无关		
for all I know	谁知道，亦未可知	get acquainted with	知道，了解；认识
for anything	无论如何	get ahead	取得进步；能储钱；不负债
for certain	肯定地，无疑地	get ahead of	越过，胜过，优于
for company	陪着，陪伴	get along	进展；相处 (with)；离开
for example (instance)	例如，举例来说	get away with	逃避惩罚（责任）
for fear (of, that)	生怕，惟恐；为防…起见	get back	回来
for free	免费	get back at	报复，报仇
for good (and all)	永久地，永远	get by	满足；过得去；勉勉强强过下去
for long	长久		
for nothing	免费，不要钱	get cold feet	失去勇气；临阵退缩；开始感到胆怯
for one thing	首先，一则；举个理由		
for oneself	为自己	get down	（从…）下来；下车；写下；咽下
for real	真的（地）；认真的（地）		
for sale	出售的，上市的	get down to	开始认真对待；认真处理
for short	简称，缩写	get even	还清欠款
for sure	确实，毫无疑问	get going	出发；开始
for the benefit of	为…的利益	get hurt	受伤
for the future	从今以后，将来	get in	进入；到达
for the moment	暂时，目前	get in on	参加
for the sake of	为了…起见	get in touch with	与…联络，与…取得联系
for the time being	暂时，目前	get into	进入；穿上（衣、鞋等）
forgive and forget	不念旧恶，不记仇	get into trouble	招致麻烦；陷入困境
free from (of)	不受…影响；免于…的	get it	弄懂
free of charge	免费的	get nowhere with sth.	对…毫无进展
fresh in sb's mind (memory)	记忆犹新	get off	（从…）下来；离开；动身
from abroad	从国外，从海外	get off the ground	成功地开始；进步；顺利进行
from head to end	从头到尾		
from end to end	从头到脚，全身		
from morning till night	从早到晚	get on	（使）上（车、马、飞机、船等）
from now on	从现在开始，今后	get on in life (the world)	发迹，出头；成功
from scratch	从头开始；白手起家	get on in years	上年纪，变老

get on one's feet (legs)	站起来；恢复信心；自立	give place to	让位于；被…所替代
get on sb's nerve	刺激神经，使某人觉得心烦	give rise to	引起，导致
get on the ball	专心做事；变机警	give sb. a big hand	向某人热烈鼓掌
get on to	联系	give sb. a break	给某人改过自新的机会
get on with	与…相处；继续	give sb. a bit (piece) of one's mind	对某人直言不讳
get one's back up	发怒		
get one's hand in	熟悉；熟练	give sb. a free hand	让某人自行处理
get (have) one's (own) way	随心所欲，想怎样就怎样	give (offer) sb. a lift	让某人搭车
get out	(使)出去；离开；取出	give sb. a hard time	给某人增添麻烦；捣蛋
get out of	从…出来，逃脱；避免	give sb. a pain	使某人讨厌；使某个烦恼
get out of bed on the wrong side	一早起床就情绪不佳；脾气不好	give sb. an advantage over	使某人占优势
		give sb. beans	处罚(责骂)某人
get out of the way	避开，让开	give sb. credit for	为…而称赞某个；把…归功于某人
get over	克服，战胜；复原		
get through to	使理解	give sb. hell	使某个受不了；狠揍(骂)某个一顿
get ready	完成		
get rid of	(使)准备好	give sb. the air (gate)	解雇某人；拒绝某人
get soaking wet	摆脱；除去；处理掉	give sb. the axe	解雇某人；开除某人
get somewhere	淋成落汤鸡	give sb. the benefit of the doubt	未有确证前宁信其无
get sth. off one's chest	取得进展		
get sth. out of one's mind (head)	把要讲的话讲出来；倾吐胸中积闷	give sb. the boot	解雇某人，开除某人
		give sb. the bucket	解雇某人，开除某人
get straight A's	取得全优成绩	give (show) sb. the (a) cold shoulder	冷淡地对待某人
get the ball rolling	开始进行某种工作		
get the blues	心情很沉重；心里很闷	give sb. the time of day	(与某人)相互问好，聊一会
get the sack	被解雇，被辞退	give up	放弃
get through	结束，完成；(电话)打通，消磨(时间)	give way to	让步；为…所代替
		glance at	看一眼，扫视，匆匆一瞥
get through to	使理解	go about	走来走去；流传
get through with	完成，成功	go after	追逐；追求
get to the bottom of	弄清…的真相，详细调查	go ahead with	继续做
get together	聚集；收集	go all the way with	完全一致，完全同意
get under control	控制住，抑制住	go along with	陪同…一起去；赞同，附和
get under way	出发；(船)启航	go around (round)	足够分配
get up	起床	go back to	返回到；追溯到
get up the nerve	鼓起勇气；放大胆子	go beyond	越出；超过，胜过
get up to	追及，赶上	go broke	破产
get used to	习惯于	go by	凭…判断；(时间等)过去；顺便走访
get well	复原		
give an account of	叙述；说明，解释	go down	下去；(价格等)跌落
give (lend) (an) ear to	倾听；注意	go Dutch	各自付账
give an eye to	留心，注意；照料	go for	被…吸引；喜欢
give away	赠送，捐赠；分发	go forward	前进；进行，进展
give back	归还	go from bad to worse	越来越坏，每况愈下
give birth to	生，产生，造成	go in for	从事，致力于；爱好；参加(竞赛等)
give credit to	相信，信以为真		
give forth	发出(声音气味等)	go in one ear and out the other	心不在焉，听不进去
give in	投降、屈服，让步；交上		
give notice	通知；预先通知…退职	go into	探究，调查
give off	放出，散出	go into business	从事商业

go on	继续；持续；发生；进行
go on the stage	当演员
go out of business	停业，歇业
go out of one's mind	精神错乱，发疯
go out of sight (view)	看不见
go out of the (one's) way	不怕麻烦；格外努力；特地
go out on one's own	独立地，凭自己的力量
go over	仔细检查；温习
go steady	求爱；成为关系相当确定的伴侣
go straight	笔直走；改过自新
go through	通过；经历；仔细检查
go through (a) channel (s)	通过必要的途径（渠道）
go through with	做完，完成
go to bed	就寝，上床
go too far	走得太远；做（说）得过分；过分
go up	增长；（物价等）上涨
go up in the world	在社会中得到更高的地位
go with	与…相配；协调；陪…一起去
go with the times	赶上时代；赶时髦
go without	没有；无需；没有…也行
go without saying	不用说，不言而喻
good for anything	能做各种工作；对一切都适用
good for nothing	毫无用处的，不中用的
grin and bear it	默默忍受痛苦；逆来顺受；咬紧牙关
grow up	长大；成长；成人
gummed tape	胶带

H

had better	还是…好，最好还是；应该（后接不带 to 的不定式）
hammer out	推敲出，设计出
hand down	传下来，传给（后代等）
hand in	交进，交上
hand out	分给，分发
handwriting (writing) on the wall	不祥之兆，凶兆
hang around	徘徊，逗留
hang on to	不挂断（电话）；坚持不去
hang up	挂断（电话）
happen on (upon)	偶然发现（碰到）
happen to	发生，落到
hard cash	硬币；现金
hard feeling	生气；怀恨，敌意

hardly ever	几乎从不；很少
have a date	有约会
have a fancy for	爱好
have a go at	试试
have a good head for	有…的才能
have a good (high) opinion of	对…评价好
have a good time	过得快活
have a hand in	参与，参加
have a rough time	吃苦，受难
have (run) a temperature	发热
have a way with	对…具有说服或影响的能力
have a word with	和…谈谈
have access to	可以到达；可以使用
have an effect on (upon)	对…有影响
have an eye for	很能鉴赏、判断
have an eye to	照看；注视
have confidence in	信任
have control over (of)	能控制
have enough of	受够了，再忍受不住了
have faith in	相信
have got to	不得不，必须
have no business to	没有权力（理由）
have no choice but to (do)	除（做）…外别无他法
have no opinion of	认为…不行，对…看法不好
have nothing to do with	与…没有关系；不跟…往来
have on	穿着，戴着
have one's cake and eat it	两者兼得（常用于否定句）
have one's hands free	手空着；没事干
have one's hands full	手头工作很忙
have one's own way	我行我素，随心所欲
have second thoughts	经过重新考虑而改变主意、看法
have seen better days	昔盛今衰，曾盛极一时
have the advantage of	占…优势
have the bell at one's feet	有机会获得成功
have to do with	与…有关系；与…有来往
have words (with)	（和…）争吵；斥责
head and shoulders above	（指智力或能力方面）远远高出；大大胜过
head for	前往
head over heels	颠倒地；匆忙地
hear from	接到…的信（电话）
hear of	听到；得知
hear oneself think	集中注意力思考
hear (listen to) reason	听从劝告
heart and soul	全心全意（地）
help oneself (to)	自取所需（食物等）
help out	帮助；帮忙完成
high time	正是该做某事的时候了
hit on (upon)	偶然碰见；忽然想到

hit the ball	成功,做得好	in addition to	除…之外
hit the ceiling	勃然大怒	in all	共计,总共
hit the nail on the head	说得中肯;做得恰到好处	in an instant	立刻,马上
hit the road	启程;上路	in appearance	看上去,外表上
hold back	退缩;隐瞒	in black and white	写在纸上;印出来
hold by	坚持	in bloom	开着花
hold down	保持住(工作等)	in brief	总之;简言之
hold off	推迟,拖延	in case of emergency	在紧急情况
hold on	继续,坚持;不挂上(电话)	in concord	和谐地
hold the line	不要挂断电话	in condition	健康状况好,身体条件适合
hold up	阻挡,使停止;抢劫;延期	in conflict with	和…冲突(相矛盾)
hold water	(论点等)站得住脚(一般用于否定句、疑问句中)	in consequence	结果,因此
		in contact with	和…接触;跟…有联系
hope for the best	乐观,从最好的方面着想	in corners (a corner)	秘密地
How about that!	好极了! 太好了!	in course of time	最后;终于;总有一天
How come?	怎么会? 为什么?	in danger (of)	有(…的)危险
hunt for (after)	寻找	in days to come	将来,此后
hurry away (off)	匆匆离去	in debt	欠债
hurry through	匆匆做完	in demand	有需要的,销路好的
hurry up	(使)赶快;赶快做完	in detail	详细地;逐条地
		in difficulties	处境困难(尤指经济上)

I

I couldn't agree (with you) more	我完全赞同你的看法	in dispute	在争论中
		in dozens	成打地(包装)
I dare say	我认为,我想	in due course	到适当的时候
I have no idea (of)	一点也不知道,听也没听说过	in earnest	认真地;郑重地
		in effect	在实行中,有效
I'll give you a buzz	我会打电话给你	in evidence	显而易见的
I'll survive	我无所谓	in excess of	多于;超过
I'll tell you what	我跟你说;我有话要告诉你	in exchange for	交换,调换
if only	但愿;要是…就好了	in existence	存在的;现存的
ill at ease	局促不安;不自在;不舒服	in fact	事实上,实际上
improve on (upon)	改进	in favor of	赞成,支持
in a bad mood	心情不好	in flower	开着花
in a bad temper	发脾气,生气	in full swing	正在全力进行;正处在高潮中
in a breeze	毫不费力地		
in a family way	受孕;怀小孩	in general	大体上,通常,一般说来
in a hurry	匆忙,立即	in good order	整齐;情况正常
in a mess	混乱;乱七八糟	in good shape	情况良好
in a minute	马上,立刻	in hand	在手中,现有的
in a moment	立即,马上	in harmony with	与…协调一致;与…相符合
in a nutshell	非常简洁地,简而言之	in haste	急速地;草率地
in a sense	从某种意义上(说)	in honor of	为庆祝,为纪念
in a way	在某种程度上;有几分	in line for	有得到…的希望,即将获得
in a while	稍后;过一会儿;不一会儿	in liquor	喝醉
in a word	总而言之,简言之	in love	恋爱中;热爱中
in addition	除此之外;并且	in low spirits	情绪低落,不高兴
		in many aspects	在许多方面
		in memory of	纪念
		in no time	很快,立刻

in one's infancy	在初期
in order	整齐,秩序井然
in particular	特别,尤其
in person	亲自
in place of	代替
in print	已出版的;(书等)在销售的,还能买到的
in progress	在进行中,正在发生
in reality	事实上,实际上
in sb's favor	对某人有利;得某人欢心
in season	盛产季节,正当时令
in shift	轮班
in spite of	尽管;不顾
in store	贮存着
in the case of	就…来说,至于
in the course of	在…过程中;在…期间
in the dark	在黑暗中;不知道,未被告知
in the end	最后,终于
in the event of	倘若,万一,如果发生
in the light of	按照,根据;从…的观点
in the long run	从长远的观点来看;终究
in the name of	以…的名义;代表
in the opinion of	据…的见解(亦作 in one's opinion)
in the red	亏损;负债
in the vicinity (of)	在…的附近;靠近
in the wake of	紧跟在…之后,紧随
in the works	正在准备(计划、进行)之中
in the world	到底,究竟(加强语气)
in time	及时
in turn	依次,轮流
in vain	徒劳,白费;无效
in vogue	正在流行,正时兴
incline to	倾向于
inclusive of	包括,连…在内
indifferent to	对…无兴趣;对…不关心
inspire confidence in sb	激起某人的信心
instead of	代替
interfere in	干涉,干预
interfere with	妨碍,打扰,干涉
involve in	卷入,陷入
itch for	渴望
It could be better	这还不够好
It could be worse	还有更糟的呢,这算可以啦
It couldn't be better	太好了
It couldn't be worse	太糟糕了
It's due tomorrow morning	明天上午要交
It's my treat	我请客
It's really nothing	真的没什么

J

Jack of all trades	万事通;杂而不专的人
join in	参加,加入;同…一起 (with)
jump at	匆匆做出(结论)
jump to a (the) conclusion	草率下结论
jump to it	赶快,立即行动
jump together	一致,符合
just about	差不多,几乎
just for the hell of it	只是为了好玩
just as	正像;正在…时候
just as well	幸运,幸好
just now	现在,眼下
just the job	正是所需要的
just the same	完全一样;还是,仍然
just too bad	太遗憾

K

keep a (the) secret	保守秘密
keep a straight face	忍不住笑出来
keep after	不断地提醒
keep an eye on	照管,照看
keep an eye out for	注意,提防
keep clear of	避开;避免
keep dark	隐瞒,保守秘密
keep from	抑制,忍住,防止
keep good time	(钟表)走得准确
keep in touch with	保持与…的接触(联系)
keep on	继续(做某事)
keep one's fingers crossed	希望,成功;祝好运
keep one's head	保持镇静,不激动
keep one's mouth shut	保持缄默;住口
keep one's word	遵守诺言、守信
keep pace with	跟…齐步前进
keep spat a distance	与某人保持相当距离;冷淡对待某人
keep silent (silence)	保持沉默,不讲话
keep the ball rolling	使(谈话等)继续下去
keep track of	记录;掌握…的线索
keep up with the Joneses	(在物质等方面)赶上富邻居
kick sth. around	从各个角度考虑(调查、讨论等)
kick the bucket	死
kill time	消磨时间;消遣
kind of	有点儿,有几分
kiss goodbye	吻别
knit up	织补;恢复;建立

knock oneself out	拼命攻读；干得筋疲力尽	let on	泄露（常用于否定句）
know a thing or two	明白整理；很有经验；精明能干	let out	放大（衣服）；放出；解散；松弛
know about	知道关于…的情况	let up	停止，中止，减缓；松弛
know of	知道	lie down	躺下休息
know sb. by name	仅知其名（未见其人）	lie idle	被搁置不用；(资金)呆滞
know sb. by sight	认得某人，跟某人面熟	lie in	在于
know the ropes	知道事情的内情、窍门、规则	light up	高兴；天晴；(使)四壁生辉
known as	以…知名；通称为	like a fish out of water	如鱼离水；感到生疏，不适应
known to	为…所知	like anything	非常；全力地
knuckle down	开始认真工作、学习	(as) like (ly) as not	很可能，多半；或许

L

lag behind	落后	line up	排队
later on	以后，后来	lined up for	想要得到（工作或服务）
laugh at	嘲笑，讥笑	little by little	一点一点地，逐渐地，慢慢地
lay aside	把…放在一起；积蓄；留作别用	live by	靠…为生
lay down	放下；铺设（铁路）	live through	度过，经受住；经历
lay off	（暂时）解雇	live to oneself	过孤独的生活
lay up	贮存，储蓄；暂停使用；（因病等）卧床（常用被动语态）	live up to	不辜负；达到预期的标准
		lock out	把…锁在外面
lead the way	引路，带路	long for	渴望
lean on	依靠，依赖	long odds	极小的可能性
least of all	最不	look about	四下环顾；四处寻找
leave alone	不管，不理会，不干扰	look after	照顾；照料；关心
leave behind	留下，忘记带走	look at	看；注视，查看
leave for	去（某地）	look back	回头看；回顾
leave no stone unturned	千方百计，想尽办法	look black	面带怒色，现愠色 (at)
leave nothing to be desired	完美无缺，尽善尽美	look blue	面现忧伤之色
leave off	停止不再使用	look down on (upon)	看不起，轻视
leave out	省去，略去；遗漏	look for	寻找；寻求
leave over	留下；剩下	look for a needle in a haystack	大海捞针
leave spin the dark	不让某人知道	look forward to	盼望；期待
leave sit-up to	由…对某事做出重要的决定[选择]	look into	调查；研究
		look like a million dollars	显得容光焕发，满面春风
leave (let) well (enough) alone	不要去管；不要弄巧成拙	look on	旁观
		look one's age	看上去和年龄相称
leave word (with)	留言	look oneself again	好像恢复了（健康）
lend itself to	有助于；适宜于	look out	留神，提防
lend oneself to	帮助，同意；鼓励，支持	look over	查看，检查；粗略地看一看
let alone	不干涉，不管；更不用说	look the other way	假装没看见
let down	使失望；放下，放低	look through	检查，审校，仔细查看
let go	放开，松手；解雇；听任	look up	（在词典、参考书中）查寻；拜访
let in	缩短衣服的尺寸	look up and down	到处搜寻
let off	不惩罚，从轻处理；放（炮、烟火等）；让…下车	look up to	尊敬，敬仰
		lose courage	丧失勇气，灰心
		lose face	丢脸，失面子
		lose ground	失利，失势
		lose heart	灰心，气馁

lose interest	对…不再兴趣 (in)	make out	填写，开列；理解，了解，辨认出
lose one's balance	跌倒；失去平稳	make reference to	提及，涉及；参考
lose one's head	失去自制；激动起来	make room for	给…让出空地方（时间）
lose one's temper	发脾气，动气	make sense	有意义；讲得通
lose one's tongue	说不出话来，开不了口	make sense of	弄懂…的意思
lose one's voice	嗓子说哑；说不出话来	make terms (with)	（与…）达成协议
lose one's way	迷路	make the best of	充分利用
lose oneself	迷路，迷失方向	make time	弥补损失的时间
lose sight of	看不见	make up	编选（谎言、故事等）；调停（纠纷等）；和解
lose time	（钟、表等）走得慢		
lose track of	失去的线索，失掉和…的联系	make up for	补偿，弥补
lots of	大量的，很多的	make up one's mind	下决心，决定
luck out	运气特好，逢凶化吉；非常幸运	man of letters	学者，文人
		mark down	标低（商品的）价目；减价；记下
luck up	走运，获得成功		

M

		mark time	原地踏步；暂缓进行
made to order	定制的，定做的	mark up	加价，涨价；把…标出
make a bid for	（拍卖中）出价买；投标	mean business	是当真的，不是开玩笑的
make a call	访问	measure up to	符合，达到（希望等）
make a deal with	与…达成协议	meddle in	干涉
make a difference	有影响；很重要	meet sb. halfway	迁就某人；和某人妥协
make a down payment	付现款	meet with	无意中碰见；偶然发现
make a fire	生火	mess up	搞乱；弄乱；弄糟
make a fuss (about)	大惊小怪；小题大做	microfiche reader	显微阅读器
make a go at it	成功，干好	mix up	混淆，搞混；混合；搞糊涂
make a hit	获得成功，很受欢迎	more and more	越来越；越来越多的
make a killing	赢得大笔钱；获得最大成功	more often than not	大半，大概；很正常
make a move	搬家，迁移	more or less	有几分，多少有点
make a night of it	痛快地玩一夜；通宵宴庆	more than once	不仅一次，好多次
make a point of	认为…是必要的；重视	move up	上升；（被）提升
make account of	重视	much the same	差不多
make an end of	结束；终止；除去		

N

make an impression (on)	给…留下印象，使感动		
make (both) ends meet	使收支相抵，量入为出	name after	（用他人或他物的名字）命名
make certain	弄清楚，确定	near at hand	在手边；在近旁
make do (with)	勉强对付，凑合着用	needless to way	不用说
make every endeavor	尽一切努力	never mind	不要紧；没关系
make for	前往，走向（亦作 head for）	next door	邻家、在隔壁
make friends with	与…交朋友，和…友好	next door to	与…相邻，在…隔壁
make fun of	取笑，嘲弄	next to	接近…的；次于…的；几乎
make it up (with)	（与…）和解（讲话）	next to no time	一会儿，很少时间
make money	赚钱	next to nothing	几乎没有
make much of	从…获得很多利益，充分利用	night after night	一夜又一夜
make on difference	无关紧要；没有差别	nine times out of ten	十之八九，常常
make one's way	前进，（靠自己的努力而）成功	no better than	几乎等于，简直是
make oneself at home	随便，无拘束	no catch	不值得买的物品，不合算的东西

no doubt	无疑地；必定	on business	因事；因公
no end in sight	无尽头	on cloud nine	欣喜若狂，极乐
no fewer than	不少于	on credit	赊（购）
no go	不行，无益，不可能	on deposit	储蓄，存
no good	没用，无益，不值得	on duty	值班，上班
no laughing matter	不是开玩笑的事	on earth	究竟，到底（用于加强语气）
no longer	不再；已不	on end	连续地，不断地；竖着
no matter	没关系，不要紧；不重要	on fire	着火；充满热情
no sooner…than	一…就	on hand	现有在手头；在近处；临近
no such thing	没有这样的事	on holiday	在休假中，在度假
no use	没用；无益	on leave	在休假
no way	无论如何，决不	on no account	决不，无论如何不
nowhere near	离…很远，远远没有，远不及	on no condition	在任何情况下都不，决不
no wonder	怪不得，难怪；不足为奇	on one's own	独立地；凭自己的力量
not a bit	一点也不，毫不	on order	已定购（尚未交货）
not a chance	不可能的	on purpose	故意地；为了
not a little	不少，许多，很	on sale	廉价出售；在减价
not all that	不那么（后接形容词或副词）	on schedule	按照预定时间，准时
not at all	一点也不	on second thought (s)	经过重新考虑，在仔细考虑以后
not that I know of	据我所知不是那样		
not to mention	不用说；更不必说	on slippery ground	处于可能犯错误的境地；拿不稳
nothing but	除了…以外什么也没有；只不过		
		on strike	在罢工
nothing to speak of	不值得谈，不要紧；几乎没有	on the ball	警惕；活跃；精力充沛；能干
		on the contrary	相反，反之

O

		on the dot	准时地
oblivious of	忘记，不注意	on the go	忙碌，活跃
odd jobs	零活，杂务	on the lookout for	寻找；注意，警戒
of a size	大小相同	on one hand	一方面
of course	当然，自然，毫无疑问	on the other hand	从另一方面来说
off and on	断断续续地，不时地（亦作 on and off）	on the safe side	安全的，万无一失
		on the side	作为兼职（副业）；额外
off colour	褪了色；气色不佳；身体不舒服	on the spot	立刻；当场
		on the verge of	接近于；濒于
off hand	立即，马上；事先无准备地	on the whole	总的看来；大体上
off one's chest	一吐为快；说出心中的话以解忧	on thin ice	如履薄冰；处境危险
		on time	按时，准时
off the cuff	无准备地；即席地；非正式地	on top of the world	幸福到极点，对一切都感到满意；成功的
off the top of one's head	即席地，没有准备地	on tour	在巡回（演出、演说）中
old boy	（招呼用语）老朋友，老兄，老弟	once in a blue moon	千载难逢，非常稀罕
		once in a while	偶尔，有时
on account of	因为，由于；为了	once or twice	一两次，有时，偶尔
on an (the) average	平均来说，一般说来	once after another	一个接一个地，挨次地
on behalf of	代表，为了	one way or another	不管怎样；想方设法
on board	在船上；上船（飞机，公用车辆）	open secret	公开的秘密
		open up	开发；吐露真情
		order of the day	议事日程；风气，习尚
		out of	缺乏；没有；由于
		out of breath	上气不接下气，喘不过气来

out of control	失去控制,不能操纵
out of date	过时的;陈旧的
out of one's mind	精神错乱,发狂
out of print	(书等)已售完的;已绝版的
out of season	已过时的;不合时宜的;已过旺季的
out of stock	缺货,已无存货
out of the blue	突然
out of the question	毫无可能的;办不到的
out of the way	不挡道;偏僻
out of this (the) world	无比优良的;非凡的;出色的
out of touch with	与…无联系
out of town	出城
out of work	失业
over and over (again)	再三,反复,屡次
over sb's head	超出某人理解力
over the left	完全不是这样,恰恰相反
owing to	由于,因为

P

pack up	把…打包;收拾(行李等)
pan out	产生特殊效果,成功;发展
pass by	从…旁经过;忽略
pass down	传递;遗传
pass out	分发,分配
pass over	不予考虑(提升或任命);不注意
pass up	拒绝,放过(机会等);不理睬
pave the way for	为…做准备工作;导致
pay attention (to)	注意,专心
pay back	偿付(借款等)
pay down	付现款,先支付(部分货款)
pay off	得到好处,收到效果;有报偿
pay one's way	自负应承担的费用;不赔本
peel off	剥去(水果的皮);撕下
pick on	挑中,选中
pick out	选出,拣出
pick up	(汽车等)中途搭人(装货);购买,买进
play a joke on	开(某人的)玩笑
play by ear	(不看乐谱)凭记忆演奏,即席演奏
play it by ear	随机应变,见机行事
play with fire	玩火,做(不必要的)危险事
point of view	观点,看法;见解

point out	指出,指明
postal order	邮政汇票(单)
pride oneself on (upon)	以…自豪,以…感到满意
print out	(电子计算机)印出(储存资料)
pull a long face	板起面孔,愁眉苦脸
pull away	(使)脱身,(使)离开
pull in	(车)进站,停靠路边
pull oneself together	振作起来;恢复镇定
pull out	拔出;驶出,开出
pull over	停在路边
pull sb's leg	戏弄某人,哄骗打趣某人
pull through	(使)渡过(难关)等;(使)恢复健康
push one's luck	在很有利的形势下作多余的冒险;希望好运持续
put an end to	结束,终止;废除
put away	把…收起来,放好;储存…备用
put forward	提出(理论、意见等)
put off	推迟;拖延
put on	穿上,戴上
put one on hold	让对方握住电话别挂断
put out	熄灭;关、扑灭;生产
put through	完成(任务、学业等);(给…)接通(电话)
put together	把…集中起来;装配
put bump	为…提供食宿,接待
put up with	容忍,忍受
puzzle out	(通过苦思)解决;推敲出
puzzle over	对…苦心思索;对…迷惑不解

Q

quarrel with	和…争吵,和…争论
queer for (about, on)	对…着了迷的
quite a bit	相当多(的)
quite a little	大量(的),相当多(的)
quite a while	一段相当长的时间
quite the contrary	恰恰相反

R

raise (lift) an eyebrow	使怀疑(惊讶)
raise the roof	大声抱怨;勃然大怒;喧闹
rather than	而不是
rough draft	草稿
read back	重述(复述)《电话原稿等》以

	便核实
read between the lines	体会言外之意
read one's mind	猜透别人的心事
read sth. in (at) one sitting	一口气坐着读完
receive high ratings	深受欢迎
reckon in	把…计算(考虑)在内
red tape	官样文章；烦琐和拖拉的公事程序
refer to	提及；参考；把…归类于
regard as	把…看作，认为…是
regardless of	不顾；不注意，不关心
registration procedures	注册手续
rely on (upon)	依靠，信任
resign oneself to	听从(于)，顺从(于)，接受(既成事实)
rest on (upon)	以…为基础；依靠
rest with	取决于，归于
result from	是…的结果；由于，起于
result in	结果，终归，导致
right along	继续地，不断地
right (straight) away	立刻，马上
right now	立刻，马上，就在此刻
right on	绝对正确，完全对
right or wrong	不管对不对；不管怎样
ring a bell	使人回忆起(某事)；听起来熟悉
ring off	挂断电话；停止讲话
ring the bell	获得成功，取得良好成绩
rip off	偷窃，抢劫
rise to one's feet	站起来(发言、祝酒等)
rough in (out)	草拟，打草稿；画…轮廓
rough it	过艰苦(简单)的生活
rub sb. the right way	讨好某人；抚慰某人
rub sb. the wrong way	惹怒某人；触犯某人
rule out	排除可能性
rummage sale	清仓大拍卖；捐赠品义卖
run a mile (from)	尽量避开(某人)
run across	不期而遇，偶然发现
run behind schedule	晚点；误点
run circles around (round)	大大胜过，远远超过
run down	撞倒；(使)人逐渐精疲力竭
run for	竞选
run into	偶尔遇见
run into the ground	把…做得过分；把…用得过度
run low	减少；短缺
run out (of)	完结；用光，耗尽
run short (of)	缺少；用完，耗尽
run up against	偶然碰见；遭遇
rush through	匆匆做完，草草完成

S

safe and sound	安全无恙
Santa Claus	圣诞老人
satisfy oneself	饱餐一顿；彻底搞清楚
save one's breath	说话也没用，因而保持缄默；免开尊口
save (one's) face	保全面子
save up	储蓄，攒(钱等)
saving your presence	恕我冒昧；您别多心
say who (you)	胡扯，瞎说
scant of	缺乏…的
scare away (off)	把…吓跑，把…吓退
school of hard knocks	经验
scoop out	舀出，取出
seal off	把…封锁起来，封住
search after (for)	探索，寻找
search me	我不知道
second childhood	老年的智力衰退时期；老年糊涂
second self	知己，心腹朋友；左右手
second to none	比谁都好，首屈一指，独一无二
see about	调查，查询
see eye to eye (with sb)	(与某个)看法一致，意见相同
see in a different light	以另一种观点来看待
see into	调查
see red	发怒，怒不可遏
see sb. off	为某个送行
see straight	看清东西
see the light (of day)	出现，问世，(书籍的)出版
see things	产生幻觉
see through	看透；看穿，识破
see to	负责，照料；注意，留心
seek after (for)	探索，追求
sell out	卖完，脱销
send for	派人去请，召唤
set an example	树立榜样(典范)
set aside	留出，拨出
set back	阻碍…的进程，耽搁
set in	到来，开始
set off	出发，动身
set one's heart at rest (ease)	使某个安心、放心
set one's heart on (upon)	决心要，很想要
set out	出发，开始
set (get, start) the ball rolling	开始活动(尤指谈话)

set the world on fire	非常成功，大出名		不妙
set to	开始认真干起来，大搞起来	snap out of it	改变精神状态，振作起来
set up	开办，设立；创立；建立	sneeze at	轻视，藐视
settle back	舒适地仰坐	so far	迄今为止
settle down	定居；(使)平静下来；专心致志于 (to)	so far, so good	到目前为止一切顺利
		so much the better	那就更好
settle for	对…感到满足，满足于	so much the worse	那就更糟
settle on	选择；决定，选定	soak to the skin	使(某人)浑身透湿
settle up	还清(欠款)；付清(账目等)	soak up	吸收，吸取
settle off	抖落，掸去；摆脱；驱除(疾病等)	soft drink	饮料
		some day	(将来)总有一天
shape up	形成；成长，进展	some time	相当长的时间
short (near) cut	近路，捷径	something of the kind	类似的事物
short of	不足，缺少	something smells fishy	有点可疑；有点靠不住
short of breath	呼吸短促，喘气	somewhat of	稍，略
show off	使显眼；炫耀；卖弄	sooner or later	迟早(总有一天)
show sb. round (around, over)	引导某个参观	sort of	有几分，稍稍
		sort out	整理，分类
show sb. the ropes	告诉某个事情的做法	spare no pains	全力以赴，不遗余力
show up	出席，到场	speak highly of	赞扬(某个)
shut down	关闭；(使)停工，(使)停业	speak one's mind	坦率地说出自己的想法
sick and tired of	(对…)十分厌烦	speak up	大声说(亦作 speak out)
sick at heart	感到不安和愁闷，忧心忡忡	speed up	(使)加快速度
sick of	对…(极)厌倦	speed limit	限速
side by side	肩并肩地；一起	spell out	详述；详加解释
side issue	枝节问题	spick and span	崭新的，整洁的
sign in	签到	split of a hurry	非常匆忙
sign off	(电台)停止广播	spring up	迅速地发生，出现
sign on	(电台)开始广播	stand a chance	有…希望(机会)
sign up	签字参加(工作、组织等)	stand back	退后，靠后站；不参与
sink in	被充分理解(领会)；留下印象	stand by	和…站在一起；支持
		stand for	代表；象征，意味着
sit back	(在紧张的活动之后)宽舒地休息	stand in for	担任…代表，代替(某人)
		stand in sb's way	阻挠某个
sit for	参加(考试等)	stand in the way of	阻挠(妨碍)(某事)
sit out	一直坐到(演说、演出等)结束；比…坐得久	stand on one's own legs	自主，自立
		stand out	突出；显眼
six of one and half-a-dozen of the other	半斤八两，差不多	standing joke	(老是被人嘲笑的)笑柄
		start from scratch	从头做起，白手起家
skim through	浏览(书、文章等)	start off	出发，离开
sleep late	(早晨)起得晚，睡懒觉	start out	出发，动身；着手进行
sleep like a log (top)	睡得很熟	stay up	不睡觉，熬夜
sleep off (away)	以睡眠消除(度过)	step aside	让路；避开；让位
sleep on (upon, over)	把(问题、决议等)推延到第二天解决，延期解决	step by step	逐步地；稳步地
		step down	走下(车等)；辞职；下台
sleep the clock around	睡 12 个小时	step off	下(车、飞机等)
slip of the pen	笔误	step out	离开，走出
slip of the tongue	失言，口误	step up	增加，加快，加紧
slip sb's mind	被某人遗忘	stick around	在附近逗留或等待
smell a rat	感到有可疑之处，感到事情	stick by (to)	坚持(意见等)；信守

stick to it	坚持下去	take it (things) easy	休息;从容,不急
stick together	粘在一起;团结起来	take it from me	相信我的话,我敢担保(亦作
stock up on (with)	储备,囤积		take my word)
stop by	(顺便)访问	take it out of	使疲乏不堪,使虚弱
stop over	作短暂访问	take measures	采取措施、行动
stop up	不就寝;睡得迟	take (make) notes	记笔记
straight talk	坦率(直爽)的谈话	take notice	注意,留心
straighten it out	澄清,解决;结算	take off	(飞机等)飞起,动身,离开;
stumble upon	偶然碰见,偶尔发现		脱下(衣帽等)
such as	像…这(样)样的;诸如…之	take on	呈现(新面貌等);雇用;接
	类的,例如		纳(乘客)
suffer from	因…遭受痛苦(不适)	take one's time	慢慢来,从容进行;拖拉
sum up	合计,总计	take one's turn	轮流
sure enough	果然,果真;确实	take over	接收,接管;接任
sure thing	当然,一定;毫无疑问的事	take part (in)	参与,参加
surface mail	平信	take place	发生;进行
sweep the country	突然风行全国	take sb's place	替代某人
sweet tooth	对甜食的喜爱	take shelter	躲避,寻求庇护
swing a deal	做成一笔交易	take the chair	就任会议主席;主持开会
swing it	装病骗人	take the consequences	承担后果
switch off	使…断路,关掉(电灯等)	take the floor	(在会上)起立发言;参加
switch on	使…接通,开动,启动		跳舞
switch through (to)	把(电话)接通	take the place of	代替
		take the plunge	冒险尝试;(经过踌躇后)采
			取果断的行动

T

		take to	开始从事于,致力于;喜爱
		take turns	依次,轮流
take a break	休息一会儿	take up	开始从事(某种职业、学
take a chance	冒险;投机(亦作 take		习等)
	chances)	talk about	谈论;讨论
take a crack at	试一试	talk down to	高人一等地对某人说话
take (a) pleasure in	以…为乐,喜欢	talk of the devil	说到某个(某个就到)
take (a) pride in	以…自豪,对…感到满意	talk off the of one's head	即席讲话,无准备地讲话
take account of	考虑;重视	talk sb. into sth.	说服某个做某事
take advantage of	利用	take sb. out of sth.	说服某个不做某事
take after	与(父母等)相像,长得像…	talk (speak) sense	说话有道理
take (an) interest in	对…感兴趣(亦作 have an	talk shop	讲有关本行的话,三句不离
	interest in)		本行
take a lot of nerve (guts)	勇敢,有胆量	team up with	与…合作;与…勾结
take by surprise	使诧异(吃惊)	tear down	拆毁;拆卸;扯下
take care of	照顾,照料;处理;负责	tell apart	辨别,区分
take charge	看管;负责 (of)	tell it like it is	说真话,如实反映情况
take courage	鼓起勇气,奋勇	ten to one	十之八九,很可能
take down	拿下,咽下;记下	tend on	服侍,招待
take effect	(药等)见效,奏效;(法规等)	thank God (goodness)	谢天谢地,幸亏
	生效	thanks to	幸亏;由于
take for	把…当作;误认为	That's it for today	今到此结束
take for granted	想当然;认为理当如此	That's neat	真棒!
take in	改小(衣服),缩短;欺骗	that's nothing new	你又说这话,没什么稀奇了
take into account	考虑到,顾及	That's too far ahead	你扯得太远了

the lion's share	较大的份额	toss and turn	辗转不能入睡
The line's busy	（电话）占线，有人在打	touch on (upon)	涉及；略为提到
the name of the game	本质的东西；事物的关键	trade in	作"…"方面的交易；以（旧
the next best	仅次于最好的		物）折价换取（同类新物）
the very same	正是这个；完全相同的（加强语气用）	true of life (nature)	逼真的；真实的
		true to one's name	名副其实
then and there	当时当地；当场；立刻	try on	试穿；试戴；试用
these days	现今，现在，目前	try out	参加（运动员、演员等的）选
think about	考虑；回想，想起		拔；试验
think aloud (out loud)	自言自语；想到就说出	tune in	收听（某电台）；收看（某
think highly of	对…评价很高；非常看重		频道）
think little of	轻视；把…看成不重要	turn a (one's) blind eye to	对…熟视无睹；假装未见
think of	有…的看法（想法）；考虑	turn a deaf ear to	对…根本不听，对…置若
think over	仔细考虑		罔闻
think poorly of	对…评价低；低估	turn down	拒绝；驳回；关小，调低
think twice	重新（仔细）考虑	turn green	妒忌
throw a wet blanket on (over)	对…泼冷水，使扫兴	turn off	关闭
		turn on	拧开，打开
throw away	扔掉，抛弃	turn one's back on (upon)	对…置之不理
throw the book at	给…以最严厉的惩罚	turn out	生产，制造；证明是；结果是
throw up one's hands	认输，失败；绝望	turn up	旋大，开大
throw up one's hands in horror	惊慌失措；束手无策	turn up one's nose at	对…嗤之以鼻，瞧不起
		twists and turns	迂回曲折
thumb through	翻查，浏览		
tie down	束缚，限制		

U

tie up with	忙于做	under age	未成年的，未到法定年龄的
time enough	还早，来得及	under consideration	在考虑中，在研究中，在讨论中
tired of	（变得）厌倦（腻烦）		
tit for tat	针锋相对	under control	在控制之下，被控制住
to a dot	正确地，恰好，丝毫不差地	under sail	扬帆；在航行中
to begin with	首先，第一；最初，开始	under sb's roof	寄住在某个人家里，受某
to date	到目前为止		人的招待
to make a long story short	长话短说，简而言之	under suspicion	被怀疑；有嫌疑
to no avail	无作用的；失败的	under the auspices of	由…主办，在…保护（赞
to one's heart's content	心满意足地；尽情地		助）下
to one's taste (liking)	合某个人的口味，中某个人的意	under the care of	在…照管下，由…管理
		under the influence	酒醉
to say nothing of	更不用说	under the weather	不舒服，有点小病；精神不佳
to say the least (of it)	至少可以这样说		
to some extent	在某种程度上	under warranty	在保修期
to tell the truth	老实说（作插入语用）	under way	进行着，在进行中；已着手
to the best of one's ability	尽全力	uniform with	与…同一形式（外貌）
to the ground	彻底地	up a (gum) tree	处于困难，进退两难；不知所措
to sb's knowledge	就某个所知		
to the contrary	与此相反的	up a stump	处境尴尬；茫然失措；困惑不解
to the minute	一分不差地，恰好		
to the point	中肯，切题	up against	面临，面对
together with	和，连同	up against it	面临极大的困难（尤指经济
too good to be true	好得令人难以置信；哪有这么好的事		

	困难)
up against the wall	在非常困难的境地,碰壁
up and coming	精力旺盛的,生气勃勃的,上进的
up and doing	忙碌的;活泼的;勤快的
up and down	到处;彻底地,完全地
up in the air	未定的,悬而未决的
up (down) sb's alley	适合某个兴趣(才能)的,为某个所熟悉(精通)的
up the wall	恼火的,狂热的,心烦意乱的
up to	正在做,从事干;胜任;该由…决定(选择)
up to date	直到现在的;现代化的,新近的
up to now (the present)	到现在为止,至今
up to the minute (moment)	最近的,最新式的
ups and downs	盛衰;成败;苦乐
upside down	颠倒,倒置地;乱七八糟地
use one's head	动脑筋,思考(常用于祈使句)
use up	耗尽,用完,使…筋疲力尽(常用于被动语态)
used to	过去常常,过去惯常

V

Valentine's Day	圣瓦伦丁节(二月十四日情人节)
vary with	随…而改变
vicious circle	恶性循环
visit with	拜访…,在…家里做客
void of	缺乏,没有
vote against	投票反对
vote down	投票否决
vote for	投票赞成
vote in (into, on, onto)	选举,选出来
vote out	选举中击败(原任者)

W

wade through	涉过(水、泥泞等);困难地通过
wait about (around)	不耐烦地等待
wait for it	等着,别慌
wait on (upon)	服侍,伺候;陪伴(来宾等)
wait out	(耐心)等到…结束
wait up for	(为…而)熬夜等候;停下来等…赶上

wake up	醒来;叫醒
walk away from	从…旁边走开,离开
walk heavy	神气活现
walk into	狼吞虎咽地吃,尽情地吃;痛骂,严斥
walk of life	职业;行业;阶层
walk on air	洋洋得意,飘飘然
walk out	退席;罢工
walk sb. off his legs (feet)	使某人做得筋疲力尽
walking skeleton	骨瘦如柴的人,皮包骨的人
ward off	避开;挡住;防止
warm up	(使)变热;预热;使兴奋,活跃
wash up	洗餐具
waste one's breath	徒费唇舌,白说
watch one's step	走路小心;谨慎行事
watch one's tongue	说话注意
wear and tear	磨损,耗损
wear away	(使)磨损;(体力、勇气)消耗殆尽
wear down	磨损,损耗;使筋疲力尽;使厌倦
wear out	穿破,用坏,用旧;使疲乏
wear well	经久耐用;持久地令人满意
weary out	使精疲力竭,使困乏
weather through	渡过(风暴、难关等),经受住
weigh on (upon) sb's mind	使某人烦恼;使某人心情沉重
well enough	很,相当;还可以
well off	生活宽容的,处境好的;幸运
wet blanket	败兴的事;扫兴的人
wet to the skin	浑身湿透
what for	为什么原因;为什么目的
what if	如果…将会怎样
what of…	有什么关系(要紧)
what though	尽管…有什么关系
what with	由于,因为
What's the point?	那有啥用?那又怎样呢?
whether or not	不管怎样;无论如何
Whichever you like	两者均可,随你挑
white lie	小小的谎话,不怀恶意的谎话
who's who	谁是谁;名人录
win by a neck (head, short head)	以些微之差得胜
win one's bread	糊口,谋生
win one's way	奋力前进(排除困难)取得成功
win out (through)	(经过困难、波折等)取得成功

wind up	上紧（钟表等的）发条；结束，完成，终止	word for word	逐字地；精确地
wipe out	擦净；消灭，毁灭	work away (at)	不停地继续工作
with a grain of salt	（演出等）大大地（成功），非常地（受欢迎）	work it	完成，做好
with a grain of salt	有保留地；不全信地	work on	继续工作；从事（某项工作）
with a light heart	心情愉快地，高高兴兴地	work one's way	（排除困难或障碍）奋力前进
with a view to	以…为目的，为了	work (one's way) through	完成
with a will	热情地，起劲的	work out	解决；算出；操练
with all one's heart	真心诚意地，十分愿意地	worry oneself	自寻烦恼，不必要地着急
with (all one's) might and main	尽全力，全力以赴地	worse and worse	越来越坏，每况愈下
		worse for wear	被用坏的；被穿破的
with flying colours	出色地，成功地	worth (sb's) while	值得（某人）花费时间（精力），合算的（亦作 worth it）
with half a heart	半心半意地，勉勉强强地		
with much ado	费尽心血，煞费苦心	wrap up	结束；解决，完成
with one accord	一致地，无异议地	write down	写下，记下
with one consent	经一致同意	write up	把…写成文；整理（笔记等）；详细报道
with one's eyed open	注意地，警惕地		
with open mouth	张着口；张口结舌地	wrong side out	表里倒置地，反面外露地
with pleasure	愉快地，高兴地；十分愿意		
with reason	有道理；合乎情理；正当地		
with reference to	关于（亦作 with regard to）		

Y

year after year	年复一年地
year by year	一年一年地，逐年
year in (and) year out	年年
You bet	当然，的确；绝对如此
You can be fined	你可能被罚款
You can say that again	我同意你的观点
You don't say!	我真意想不到；有这样的事！
You said it.	你说对了，我完全同意。
You're all set.	你一切准备就绪了。
You are connected.	已经接通了。
You're not putting me out at all.	一点也不麻烦。
You're telling me!	还要你告诉我！我早就知道了！

with respect to	涉及，关于
within a stone's throw of	离…一箭之远，在…附近；距离…不远
within (easy) reach (of)	在…附近；距离…不远
within limits	在一定范围内；适度地
within one's means	量入为出
within touch of	在…的附近；…能达到的
without a break	不间断地，不停顿地；不休息地
without a hitch	顺利无阻地；成功地
without (any) loss of time	立即，马上
without book	凭记忆；无根据地
without end	无穷无尽的，永久的
without fail	必定，务必
without limit	无限度；无限制的
without much (more) ado	不再哆嗦；立即，干脆
without reference to	不论，不顾；与…无关
without regard to	不考虑，不注意，不顾
without respect to	不管，不顾虑

Z

zero hour	关键时刻，紧急关头
zing up	使有生气；给…增添风趣
zonk out	很快入睡

Part Ⅵ Medical English Wordlist

医学英语词汇表

ache	疼痛	clinic	医务室,门诊部,临床
acid	n. 酸,迷幻药 adj. 酸的,讽刺的,刻薄的	cold	伤风感冒
		color blindness	色盲
activate	vt. 刺激,激活 vi. 有活力	complex	adj. 复杂的,合成的,综合的 n. 联合体
acupuncture	针灸		
allergy	过敏症	component	n. 成分 adj. 组成的,构成的
ambulance	救护车	concentrate	v. 集中,浓缩
analyze	vt. 分析,分解	conclude	v. 结束,终止,决定,作出结论 vt. 推断,断定,缔结,议定
ankle	踝		
antibiotic	抗生素	consulting room	候诊室
approach	n. 接近,逼近,走近,方法,步骤,途径,通路 vt. 接近,动手处理 vi. 靠近	contact lenses	隐形眼镜
		contrast	vt. 使与…对比,使与…对照 vi. 和…形成对照 n. 对比,对照,(对照中的)差异
approximate	adj. 近似的,大约 v. 近似,接近,接近,约计		
		cough	咳嗽
area	n. 范围,区域,面积,地区,空地	cramp	抽筋
		criterion	n. (批评判断的)标准,依据,规范
aspirin	阿司匹林		
assay	n. 化验 v. 化验	culture	n. 培养,培养物
assess	vt. 估定,评定,测定	data	n.datum 的复数,[计] 资料,数据
available	adj. 可用到的,可利用的,有用的,有空的,接受探访的		
		define	vt. 定义,详细说明
baseline	n. 基线	demonstrate	vt. 示范,证明,论证 vi. 示威
bleed hemorrhage	出血		
bronchitis	支气管炎	design	n. 设计,图案,花样,企图,图谋,(小说等的)构思,纲要 v. 设计,计划,谋划,构思
bruise/wound	伤痕		
burn	烧伤		
capsule	胶囊	detect	vt. 察觉,发觉,侦查,探测 v. 发现
cavity	龋齿洞,腔,窝,窝洞		
channel	n. 海峡,水道,沟,路线 vt. 引流,引导,开导;信道,频道	diagnosis	诊断
		diarrhea	腹泻
		diet pill	减肥药
check over/physical exam	体检	dietician	营养师
chest	胸部	digestive	消化药
pediatrician	小儿科医生	disorder	n. 杂乱,混乱,无秩序状态 vt. 扰乱,使失调,使紊乱
chill	受寒		
chronic	慢性的,延续很长的	distribute	vt. 分发,分配,散布,分布,

	分类,分区 v. 分发	induce	vt. 劝诱,促使,导致,引起,感应
dizzy	头晕		
doctor's office	诊所、医务办公室	infect	vt. 传染,感染
doctor's order (advice)	医嘱	infection	传染
donor	n. 捐赠人,供体 n.[化]原料物质	infirmary	(学校、教养所)医院、医务室
dose	n. 剂量,(一)剂,(一)服 v.(给…)服药	inflammation	n. 炎症,发炎
		inhibit	抑制,约束,[化][医]抑制
dose/dosage	剂量	initial	adj. 最初的,初始的
drugstore/pharmacy	药房		n. 词首大写字母
emergency room	急诊室	injection	打针
estimate	n. v. 估计,估价,评估	injury	n. 伤害,侮辱
euthanasia, mercy killing	安乐死	in-patient	住院部
evaluate	vt. 评价,估计,求…的值 v. 评价	insomnia	失眠
		insulin	n. 胰岛素
expose	vt. 使暴露,受到,使曝光 v. 揭露	intense	adj. 强烈的,剧烈的,热切的,热情的,激烈的
extract/pull out	拔牙	intern	实习医生
eye doctor (oculist, ophthalmologist)	眼科医生	internal medicine	内科
		internal organs	内脏
factor	n. 因素,要素,因数,代理人	intervene	vi. 干涉,干预,插入,介入,(指时间)介于其间 v. 干涉
fever	发热		
fraction	n. 小部分,片断,分数	involve	vt. 受累,包括,牵涉,使陷于
function	n. 官能,功能,作用,职责,典礼,仪式,[数]函数;vi.(器官等)活动,运行,行使职责	isolation	隔离病房
		itch	痒
		knee	膝
		lesion	n. 损害,身体上的伤害
gene	n.[遗传]因子,[遗传]基因	major	n. 主修课,专业,成年人,大调 adj. 主修的,成年的,大调的 vi. 主修
general practitioner	全科医生		
generate	vt. 产生,发生		
gum	牙龈	malfunction	功能失调
gynecologist	妇科医生	mediate	v. 仲裁,调停,作为引起…的媒介,居中调停
Head nurse	护士长		
health insurance card	健康保险卡	medical instruments	医疗仪器
heart attack	心脏病发作	medium	n. 媒体,方法,媒介 adj. 中间的,中等的,半生熟的
hepatitis	肝炎		
high blood pressure	高血压	membrane	n. 膜,隔膜
house call	出诊	metabolism	新陈代谢
hurt	撞伤,痛	mixture	合剂
identify	vt. 识别,鉴别,把…和…看成一样;v. 确定	molecular	adj.[化]分子的,由分子组成的
impact	n. 碰撞,冲击,冲突,影响,效果 vt. 挤入,撞击,压紧,对…发生影响	monitor	n. 班长,监听器,监视器,监控器 vt. 监控;v. 监控
		multiple	adj. 多样的,多重的 n. 倍数,若干 v. 成倍增加
incubate	vt. 孵卵		
indicate	vt. 指出,显示,象征,预示,需要,简要地说明	muscular	adj. 肌肉的,强健的
		nausea	恶心,反胃,作呕
indigestion	消化不良	nearsighted	近视
individual	n. 个人,个体 adj. 个别的,单独的,个人的	normal	n. 正规,常态, adj. 正常的,正规的,标准的

nuclear	adj. 细胞核的；细胞核的，中心的	receptor	n. 接收器，感受器，受体
obtain	vt. 获得，得到	region	n. 区域，地方，（世界上某个特定的）地区，（艺术，科学等的）领域，（大气，海水等的）层
old folk remedy	民间药方		
onset	n. 发作，攻击，进攻，有力的开始，肇端	release	n. 释放，让渡，豁免，发行的书，释放证书 vt. 释放，解放，放弃，让与，免除，发表 n. 版本，发布
operation-room	手术室		
ophthalmology	眼科		
outcome	n. 结果，成果		
out-patient	门诊部	require	vt. 需要，要求，命令
overall	adj. 全部的，全面的	resident doctor	住院医生
over-the-counter medicine	普通药	respective	adj. 分别的，各自的
participate	vi. 参与，参加，分享，分担	respiratory system	呼吸系统
pathway	n. 路，径	respond	v. 回答，响应，作出反应 vi. 有反应
pediatrics	小儿科		
period	n.（妇女的）经期，月经	reveal	vt. 展现，显示，揭示，暴露
periodical inspection	定期健康检查	rheumatism	风湿
pharmacist	药剂师	scan	v. 细看，审视，浏览，扫描 n. 扫描
phase	n. 阶段，状态，相，相位；v. 定相	score	n. 得分，乐谱，抓痕，二十，终点线，刻痕，账目，起跑线 vt. 把…记下，刻画，画线，获得，评价 vi. 记分，刻痕，得分 血清
physician	内科医生		
positive	adj. 肯定的，实际的，积极的，绝对的，确实的 adj. 正的；阳的；原级的		
		serum	血清
potential	adj. 潜在的，可能的，势的，位的 n. 潜能，潜力，电压	serum	n. 浆液，血清，免疫血清，树液
powder	粉状药	site	n. 地点，场所，遗址 vt. 定…的地点 n. 站点
prescription	处方		
previous	adj. 在前的，早先的	sleeping pill	安眠药
primary	adj. 第一位的，主要的，初步的，初级的，原来的，根源的	smallpox	天花
		sore throat	喉咙痛
prior	adj. 优先的，在前的 n. 预先 adv. 在…前 adv. 在…以前 (to)	source	n. 来源，水源，消息来源，原始资料，发起者，源，源极
		specific	n. 特效药，细节；adj. 详细而精确的，明确的，特殊的，特效的，[生物]种的
private practitioner	开业医师		
private ward	头等病房		
procedure	n. 程序，手续	stomach	腹部
process	n. 过程，作用，方法，程序，步骤，进行，推移 vt. 加工，处理	strain	扭伤
		strain	n. 过度的疲劳，紧张，张力，应变 vt. 扭伤，损伤 v. 拉紧，扯紧，（使）紧张，尽力
protein	n.[生化]蛋白质 adj. 蛋白质的		
psychiatrics	神经病学	stress	n. 重压，逼迫，压力，重点，着重，强调，重音 vt. 着重，强调，重读
psychiatrist	精神病医生		
range	n. 山脉，行列，范围，射程 vt. 排列，归类于，使并列，放牧；vi. 平行，延伸，漫游		
		structure	n. 结构，构造，建筑物 vt. 建筑，构成，组织
ratio	n. 比，比率，[财政]复本位制中金银的法定比价	superintendent of nurses	护士长
		surgeon	外科医生
react	vi. 起反应，起作用，反抗，起反作用	surgery	外科
		survive	v. 幸免于，幸存，生还，存活

swollen	肿	color blindness	色盲
symptom	n. 症状，征兆	contact lenses	隐形眼镜
table/pill	片剂	psychiatrics	精神病学
target	n. 目标，对象，靶子	euthanasia, mercy killing	安乐死
tartar	牙石	injection	打针
terminally ill	病入膏肓	periodical inspection	定期健康检查
test	化验	health insurance card	健康保险卡
the flu	流行性感冒	children's doctor (pediatrician)	小儿科医生
therapy	n. 治疗	eye doctor (oculist, ophthalmologist)	眼科医生
throw up, vomit	呕吐		
thumb	拇指	surgeon	外科医生
tissue	n. 薄的纱织品，薄纸，棉纸，[生]组织，连篇	gynecologist	妇科医生
		private practitioner	开业医师
toothache	牙痛	general practitioner	全科医生
Traditional Chinese Medicine (TCM)	中医	intern	实习医生
transplant	v. 移植，移种，移民，迁移 n. 移植，被移植物，移居者	pharmacist	药剂师
		sore throat	喉咙痛
		symptom	症状
tumor	瘤，肿瘤；赘生物；肿胀：肿胀的部分	test	化验
		check over/physical exam	体检
ulcer	溃疡	doctor's order (advice)	医嘱
vaccine	疫苗	internal medicine	内科
vary	vt. 改变，变更，使多样化 vi. 变化，不同，违反	cold	伤风感冒
		indigestion	消化不良
versus	prep. 对（指诉讼，比赛等中），与…相对	ophthalmology	眼科
		nearsighted	近视
visual	adj. 看的，视觉的，形象的，栩栩如生的	pediatrics	小儿科
		smallpox	天花
vitamin	维他命	prescription	处方
volume	n. 卷，册，体积，量，大量，音量	medical instruments	医疗仪器
		physician	内科医生
vomit	呕吐	psychiatrist	精神病医生
ward	病房	resident doctor	住院医生
wrist	腕	dietician	营养师
yellow fever	黄热病	superintendent of nurses	护士长

Hospital and Medicine 医院与医学术语

		ache	疼痛
		cough	咳嗽
		fever	发热
doctor's office	诊所、医务办公室	toothache	牙痛
clinic	医务室	hurt	撞伤，痛
infirmary	（学校、教养所）医院、医务室	bleed hemorrhage	出血
diagnosis	诊断	stomach	腹部
operation-room	手术室	thumb	拇指
drugstore/pharmacy	药房	allergy	过敏症
internal organs	内脏	bruise/wound	伤痕
surgery	外科	chill	受寒
respiratory system	呼吸系统	diarrhea	腹泻
the flu	流行性感冒	malfunction	功能失调
high blood pressure	高血压	infection	传染

vomit	呕吐	antibiotic	抗生素
nausea	恶习	digestive	消化药
rheumatism	风湿	mixture	合剂
yellow fever	黄热病	sleeping pill	安眠药
vaccine	疫苗	capsule	胶囊
over-the-counter medicine	普通药	vitamin	维他命
old folk remedy	民间药方	powder	粉状药
gum	牙龈	diet pill	减肥药
ward	病房	table/pill	片剂
isolation	隔离病房	dose/dosage	剂量
in-patient	住院部	Traditional Chinese Medicine (TCM)	中医
consulting room	候诊室		
ambulance	救护车	acupuncture	针灸
chest	胸部	tartat	牙石
swollen	肿	cavity	腔，窝，窝洞
wrist	腕	head nurse	护士长
knee	膝	terminally ill	病入膏肓
heart attack	心脏病发作	throw up, vomit	呕吐
ankle	踝	sweats	发汗
burn	烧伤	night sweats	盗汗
cramp	抽筋	sneeze	打喷嚏
strain	扭伤	hiccup	打嗝
metabolism	新陈代谢	low back pain	腰疼
dizzy	头晕	throbbing, colic, radiating, crampy, dull, piercing, prickling pain	一跳一跳地、绞，放射，痉挛，钝，刺，戳，针扎似的疼痛
itch	痒		
hepatitis	肝炎		
ulcer	溃疡	inhale	吸气
bronchitis	支气管炎	exhale	呼气
insomnia	失眠	difficulty in breathing	呼吸困难
serum	血清	irregular pulse	脉搏不规则
extract/pull out	拔牙	blood glucose	血糖
cavity	龋洞	cholesterol	胆固醇
private ward	头等病房	lipid	血脂
out-patient	门诊部	diabetes	糖尿病
emergency room	急诊室	hypertension	高血压
house call	出诊	hyperglycemia	高血糖
aspirin	阿司匹林	hyperlipidemia	高血脂